# Biomedical Ethics

KENNETH VAUX

# Biomedical Ethics

*Morality for the New Medicine*

**HARPER & ROW, PUBLISHERS**
New York, Hagerstown, San Francisco, London

The original material for Chapter 7, "Controlling Man," was published in the *Journal of the Medical Association of Georgia*, December 1970, and has been expanded in this book.

Acknowledgment is made to the following for permission to include copyrighted materials:

*Journal of the American Medical Association* for selection from "A Definition of Irreversible Coma" by Henry Beecher et al. Copyright © 1968 by the American Medical Association.

Random House, Inc. for selections from *Gideon* by Paddy Chayefsky. Copyright© 1962 by Random House, Inc.

First HARPER & ROW PAPERBACK edition published 1976.

*Designed by C. Linda Dingler*

**Library of Congress Cataloging in Publication Data**

Vaux, Kenneth.
  Biomedical ethics; morality for the new medicine.
  Includes bibliographical references.
  1. Medical ethics.  2. Medicine and religion.
I. Title. [DNLM: 1. Ethics, Medical.  W50 V385b 1974]
R724.V35      174'.2      73–18879
ISBN 0–06–068857–2

76 77 78 79 80 10 9 8 7 6 5 4 3 2 1

# Contents

*Preface*                                                           vii

Introduction: The Question of Man                                    ix

Part One: The Traditions of Medical Ethics                            1

  1. The Hippocratic Tradition                              3
  2. The Religious Traditions: Jewish, Arabic, Catholic, Prot-
     estant, and Marxist                     10
  3. The Neuremberg Tradition                               26

Part Two: A Model for Decision-making                                35

  4. Sources of Ethical Insight                             37

Part Three: Modern Designs and Transformations                       47

  5. Generating Man                                         49
  6. Rebuilding Man                                         69
  7. Controlling Man                                        85
  8. Immortalizing Man                                      96

Postscript: The Future of Man: They Shall Be Like
Gods . . .                                                          111

## vi    Contents

*Notes*                                      114

*Glossary*                                   129

*Index*                                      133

# Preface

This book emerges from several years' struggle to appropriate in a legitimate way the insights and values of religious faith into the complex clinical decisions of medical ethics. Working day by day with physicians and scientists in one of the world's great medical centers has made it clear that this range of problems is perhaps the most difficult yet to challenge the mind and heart of man. At the same time his survival depends on their solution. The patients, nurses, chaplains, scientists, and physicians of the Texas Medical Center in Houston have been my teachers. The humane vision of Richard T. Eastwood, Ph.D., the center's executive director, and the medical skills and human commitments of colleagues Harry Lipscomb, M.D., and Carlos Vallbona, M.D., have guided me, by example, into this area of concern. This study is dedicated to them and to the magnificent generation of medical students who now make ready to minister to their fellowman. These men and women, so well equipped by advanced science and technology, are at the same time incapacitated by an ethical wisdom insufficient to their task. The Oreon E. Scott lectureship at the Graduate School of Phillips University provided the forum where these issues could be explored with provocative feedback. To Dean Dan Joyce and the Enid, Oklahoma, community I express sincere thanks.

*Houston, Texas*                                    KENNETH VAUX

# Introduction: The Question of Man

Health is a vital concern of every human being. If we look at the spectrum of experience that we call disease, we see an ever-increasing quantum transferred from the realm of unknown etiology and cure to the area of scientific understanding and technical management. Because of this we have a compelling interest in the forces that contribute to, or detract from, health, and we are engaged in the process of transforming the values which effect our well-being as persons and communities. Most are interested in natural foods and simple lifestyles. The variety of human potential movements, encounter groups, and other growth experiences witness a quest for self-knowledge and interpersonal awareness. Our generation seeks social and political forms where human possibilities are maximized and not subverted. We want a recovery of harmony in the ecosphere where self and environment abide cooperatively rather than being juxtaposed in subject-object domination. In all these efforts our concern is to enhance those forces that build up human health and ward off those which destroy. In this sensate age it is probable that most personal habits, sociopolitical formations, spiritual experiments, and certainly most technological acts are established in pursuit of the goal of health.

It is this quest that leads us into profound moral crisis.[1] The ultimate implication of this quest for well-being is a view that sees all disease, debilitation, and even death as inimical to man's nature and his possibility. His life urge confronts with great intensity the perennial boundaries of existence. Pain cannot be endured, and a pleasure-seeking generation must also be a pill-popping generation. Death itself becomes an affront to be cosmetized and masqueraded.

The quest for health and the appropriate prerequisite values is at once a profoundly personal and detached venture. The first heart transplant, for example, both struck the center of our existence and titillated the imagination. It reminded us that we too must face bodily deterioration and death, quite possibly from cardiac failure. Our incurable fascination with the new and incredible also led us to follow this and other medical breakthroughs. The existential interest sent thousands of new "joggers" trudging earth's highways and byways. The detached fascination asked, "What will medicine do next?" or "How feasible is a brain transplant?" Medical or health ethics is at once a subject of intense personal concern, gathering to itself the hopes and fears of life and death, and a theoretical intrigue regarding the shape of the yet unknown future.

Any balanced treatment for medical ethics must hold together these two elements of personal drama and theoretical analysis. A responsible treatment will also bring together the deepest philosophical and theological understandings of man and the practical dynamics of human decision. This short book will seek to maintain this delicate tension.

The book is written for laymen as well as professionals in the health fields. It seeks to show how profound decision-making crisis implicit in this area can be submitted to ethical analysis and how a reasonable mode of rendering choice can be made. As in most books in medical ethics, my central problem is to discern the kind of question we are dealing with. I disagree with arguments which suggest that the crises of biomedicine can be reduced to economic,[2] biopolitical,[3] or even philosophical and utilitarian formulation.[4] The issues demand theological analysis. They are issues of ultimate consequence concerning the profound dimensions of human nature and destiny. The issues are therefore too important to be left to the experts and too searching to be reduced to superficial analysis.

An initial question we face is that of the meaning of human value under the impact of technology. Decisions that need to be made day by day in hospitals and clinics of a medical center are always both particularly immediate and profoundly universal. A specific clinical decision to sustain at great cost in a bubble a child born with no immunological system, for example, reflects a generalized value commitment of a culture. My work in recent years has been with physicians, interns, residents, and medical students who, in the agony of handling medical crisis day by day, slowly develop a moral *modus operandi* within which they act. To come to a working understanding of the sanctity of life delicately balanced in the personal and corporate dialectic is a continuing challenge. In the clinical settings of modern teaching hospitals the constant weight of human anguish, combined with the ever-present fact of death which is the refutation of not only our life urge but the biomedical commitment as well, conspires to create an insensitivity toward persons and a devaluation of human dignity.

A medical student reported one small vignette in this desensitizing process. He repeatedly tried to enroll in an animal surgery elective. He was thwarted several times. "The seminar is too full"; "It is canceled"; "You are not ready for it," he was told. He came to his ob-gynecology rotation and found himself the only doctor one night when a woman having just given birth began to hemorrhage. He used the scalpel and suture for the first time. He worked slowly and carefully. It took him two hours to complete the job. The resident finally arrived and had to redo the repair, sharing with him the news that quick, deliberate sutures are least painful. After this traumatic instance he demanded the animal surgery elective. In the class he asked the instructor if he could sew the head back on a dog. "Don't touch that dog," he was told. "He is too valuable."

The following is an excerpted verbatim of a conversation with an active internist:

. . . The curious paradox is that medical students come to our medical school imbued with a spirit of altruism, kindness, humanity, the dignity of man and the intrinsic right of every individual of a fair shake in health care.

Somewhere along the line, because of training programs or by the very nature of the beast of medical education, the students, if they don't lose these values, they are at least so sufficiently repressed that they never again enter the level of consciousness. Two or three known factors along with many others we don't yet understand contribute to this. It is abundantly clear that medical education with high tuition in private schools such as ours is a process which generates a significant indebtedness for a young man. By the time he has completed his training one of his first motivations is the acquisition of monies to repay his indebtedness. I should add that at least fifteen enlightened nations I know of, including the one we consider unenlightened just south of us called Mexico, have had the prescience for the last forty years to subsidize medical education. In exchange for that the *quid pro quo* they ask is public service. This recruitment forms a National Health Service corps of young Mexican medical graduates. First of all, our students are hampered by a significant economic encumbrance when they finish school, so there is a strong motive to accumulate money.

The second fact that may contribute to this value change is that young men are exposed in very intensive ways to human misery in such an overwhelming dose that it's difficult for even the most humane individual not to become inured in some way to human suffering. In fact, this could be itself the subject of significant research because it may well be that it is not a perverse turn-off mechanism but a protective turn-off mechanism to guard the ego and the mental stability of the young doctors. I can remember as a chief medical resident on a sixty-bed ward I lost five to ten patients every night and was up almost all night long virtually every night. I was living on about two hours' sleep. You can't function very long at this state without it either doing something to you or you having to do something to yourself to protect your ego and your strength. I'm not so certain that our medical education needs to be as inconsiderate as that.

A third mechanism which may work to challenge the basic faith of young physicians in human dignity is that medicine is tending toward a scientific technology as opposed to a humane art. The men from whom they learn the practice of medicine all too frequently see themselves as technicians rather than healers. Modern medicine has of necessity become an advanced scientific enterprise. The challenge today is to infuse this with humanistic commitment.

Our intense specialized disease orientation combines with an increased technology so that the patient is lost sight of. Very few medical publications deal with patients, most all of them deal with diseases. Though physicians may genuinely wish to keep sight of the patient, the sophistication of the technology available to many physicians is so great that the patient is of secondary importance. Practice focuses on killing bacteria in the bloodstream, curing septicemias or removing the disease from the person in the surgical sphere. Pediatrics has kept a modicum of humanity because the patient himself is like a veterinary patient and the doctor is forced to deal with the third party, the great advocate, the mother. In that unique position she interjects her own basic humanity into the situation. Generally when a patient goes to a physician as a free agent, there are very few protective mechanisms for his ego strength and nothing to protect his rights. The analogous situation in technology is to take your television set in for repair. You do not know the intricacies of diagnosis and repair. You are totally at the mercy of this man's conscience, his good will, his ethical and moral sense. This is not to say that my colleagues are being indemnified or villified, but the fact remains that patients in America are angry over the type of health care they are receiving, and I feel justifiably so, and have said so publicly and frequently.

The final point has to do with the type of men we admit to medical school. In the last fifteen years we have emphasized technological skill and the ability of a young person to know physics, physical chemistry, math, and the physical sciences as factors in selection. Our emphasis on choosing scientifically trained, quantitatively oriented individuals may have brought into medicine a group of people uniquely unsuited to think on affairs of the spirit and the heart. In my dealing with engineers and physical scientists in the last few years, the imponderables of the human biological system are just not something that is part of their ken. They are black box people. In the medical enterprise the profit motive; the effect of constant exposure to pain and death; technology's intrusion into patient care; the personal qualities of today's doctors and students—all these factors contribute to a general depreciation of the value of human worth.

The activity of biomedicine raises acutely the question of the nature of man. The tendency to relate human being to the animal world from which he emerges is one tendency. Numerous studies in the field of comparative ethology, anthropology, and zoology are relevant at this point.[5] The inadequacy of this literature is found in its essential evasion of the unavoidable reflective question that human being continually asks. The question of man concerning his own nature and destiny, writes Abraham Heschel, is one that is unsatisfied with exhaustive descriptions in terms of his animality or facticity.

The search for self-understanding is a search for authenticity of essence, a search for genuineness not to be found in anonymity, commonness and unremitting connaturality.[6]

At the other end of the spectrum, man's nature is compared to, or contrasted with, the machine. Man's nature, it is argued, can be explained by mathematical models and his behavior by mechanical modes.

As we ponder the basic question of how man is changed through biomedicine, we immediately confront the impact of technology. One may question whether contemporary man shapes his future with his technology or is shaped by his technology for some undesignated future. Serious debate on this issue now wages in the planning divisions of the space programs of the United States and the Soviet Union. Should we alter and transform man to meet the challenges of space exploration, or should we fabricate android systems to simulate human intelligence and function for those tasks? The problem is framed in a similar way by Dr. Jose Delgado, the brain physiologist. He hints in his writing that the mind of man must be technologically or chemically altered to meet the rigors of the "psychocivilization" we have created. Should we remake man to be at home in the environment that technology demands, or should we change the environment to suit man? While some call for ecological and population intervention, other scientists and politicians say that we should work to enhance man's adaptability to an increasingly toxic environment and congested world populace. Gas masks and geodesic domes covering cities are to be preferred over a return to the hardships of a simple relationship to the land. Shall man shape his future or be shaped by his future? This looms as one of the most challenging problems of the last decades of this century.

In this book I propose to survey a continuum of situations in the areas of human health where decisions are required. In all of these situations the ethical challenge is heightened because technology is involved. I agree with Hans Jonas when he notes that the nature of human action has changed because of the novel powers of modern technology. A man today does not make decisions as a romantic, rugged individual in a pristine environment. His active being is augmented by technologies which are more than mere extensions. They interpenetrate and interact with his personality. The environment is electrified and technicized, no longer raw nature in a way where strict causality could be prescriptive. In ethical planning and decision-making today, agency is usually complicated by technology.

Many artifacts now replace, augment, or extend the acting human person. They enlarge or limit his functioning and the change he makes on the environment. To make a meaningful valuation of human decision-making, man must be seen as an organismic unity with these technological extensions. We stand today at the end of an era that viewed nature in mechanical terms. Man as machine *(L'Homme Machine)*[7] is the prevailing perception of our time. This is precisely the reason that we have great difficulty in establishing an ethical context for health problems and fail to understand the dynamics and ramifications of moral decisions in the biomedical sphere.

Our problem is complicated by the fact that value orientations in this late sensate, technological age are skeptical, agnostic, and unclear. We now realize that our normative disciplines are increasingly incapable of bearing insight into problems of medical ethics. We simply do not know how to think ethically about man in dynamic life situations complicated by technology. The value sciences—philosophical ethics, moral theology, and theological ethics—all approach man in his pretechnological simplicity or in philosophic abstraction. Hans Jonas has shown how in our constitutive human history

action on non-human things did not constitute a sphere of authentic ethical significance. Ethical significance belonged to the direct dealing of man with man . . . . all traditional ethics is anthropocentric.[8]

We talk about the concepts of human nature, the qualities of willing the good or the destructive, but we seldom rise to the level of considering values operationally in the concrete situations where decisions are required. We have difficulty weaving the dynamic human qualities of hope, pain, suffering, and joy into a normative frame. The theological sciences have erred in their all-embracing search for a concept of human nature that is somehow transcendent of all particular men. In focusing ethical scrutiny on the act in isolation from its network of intrication and implication and its natural and technological aspect, the philosophic tradition of ethics also leaves us floundering for value insights in a technological society.

It may well be that philosophy and theology are correct and wise in shunning this profound task today. Perhaps philosophy is right to concern itself with logical and linguistic consistency within a *given* frame of reference. Perhaps its proper task is analyzing the meaning of language. Perhaps theology is becoming properly humble by forsaking its former hegemony and refocusing its energy on the quest for personalistic meaning. Certainly the church regains some semblance of servitude as it forfeits the ethical absolutism that so frequently forced moral legalisms in the past.

If this is true, then we urgently need a new discipline that will explore the new kinds of problems implicit in the technological advance. This new discipline perhaps might be an interdisciplinary quest for the structures of responsibility. This endeavor must encompass the wisdom of classic humanistic insight, plain common sense, and a lively new study of the future. It will involve the normative, descriptive, and predictive disciplines. Van Potter reaches in this direction when he calls for the discipline of "Bioethics."

This study is also a search for that new discipline. It is a search for normative guidelines in decision-making situations where some man-technology union or interface is involved. My thesis contends that ethical insight comes from three sources. The value of man's life based on human dignity and the quality of human nature is one source. From the theological heritage we affirm a dignity that man receives from beyond himself. Man has value and is to be valued as a man. From the future we affirm man's possibility. These principles from behind, within, and beyond are the roots which grow together to form an estimate of man, an axial strength on which to anchor guiding values. This truth about man also offers concrete, practical insight for decision-making.

A synopsis of history shows us how far we have come. Technology began its entree into human activity long ago. When primitive man first used a club to smash his enemies' skull, it was an act of different moral quality than injuring him in hand-to-hand struggle. Although the instrument is not responsible, of course, it did enhance man's power, thus changing the ethical dynamics. Technologies were created to enhance manual activity: the hammer, the sophisticated tools and machines, the factory. Technologies then came to extend the activities of communication, persuasion, and coercion: the Greek theater, the loudspeaker, electronic media. Then the rational, decision-making functions of man were joined and empowered by new technologies: the depressants and the stimulants of the central nervous system, the computers. Then finally, the vital organismic activities of man were augmented: the artificial organs, the biocybernetic devices. Slowly but surely, nearly every human facility and activity finds itself intricated with some artifact, some technology. The interaction, interface, or coupling of man and technology subtly distorts the dynamics of moral situations. The context blows its proportions so that boundaries defy delineation. Hidden persuaders in advertising may actually have the same ethical consequence as a situation of direct coercive brainwashing. We thought the moral culpability of pulling the lever on the bomb hatch of the Enola Gay was somehow less than strangling the enemy soldier with our hands. Spilling sulphur into the air or mercury into the river did not have the moral stigma of dropping arsenic in your husband or wife's coffee. Yet the acts were equally damaging and lethal despite the distance and time lag between action and result. Added to this is the anonymity and impersonal nature of secondary and tertiary relatedness. The moral dynamics of the ancient

Egyptian slave master were more overt than the stockholder of a corporation that likewise mistreated Chicanos on a Florida citrus farm.

We are just now entering an age wherein we can perceive moral responsibility for acts, personal and corporate, which injure fellowmen, however subtly and indirectly this harm is inflicted through the instrumentality of our technology. To unravel the dynamics of responsiveness and responsibility and discern the patterns of ethical decision-making and planning is the purpose of this book.

The argument will be developed in four parts. We must begin with a discussion of the traditions of medical ethics which contribute to a contemporary value system. The contributions of Hippocratic, religioethical, and Neuremberg traditions will be weighed. This section will conclude with a synthesis designed to be a contemporary frame of reference.

A model of decision-making will then be proposed within which the sources of ethical insight will be located. Here we will examine traditional sources, i.e., those insights that flow from memory, tradition, experience, and revelation. We will consider common sense, conscience, and collective conscience, those basic humanistic insights that proceed from common intelligence and goodwill. Then, we will explore the power of consequential insight: that predictability, both moral and technological, which tells us what will happen if we do something—before we do it. The final part of the book will deal with selected problems. Here we will survey a number of concrete situations where human vitality, under the impact of technology, is confronted with the imperative to decide and plan. The series of profound problems of health ethics emerge along the life cycle spectrum. We will organize the exploration around the topics of generating, rebuilding, controlling, and immortalizing man. A case study will seek to convey the clinical practicality and philosophical depth in each area.

# PART ONE

---

## The Traditions of Medical Ethics

---

# 1. The Hippocratic Tradition

To understand the contemporary ethos that shapes medical decision-making we must recall the wisdom of the Hippocratic tradition. The view of professional etiquette and covenantal responsibility embodied in the code deeply informs the rigorous value system of today's practitioner of medicine. "There is no profession," says Paul Ramsey, "that comes close to medicine in its concern to inculcate, transmit and keep in constant repair its standards governing the conduct of its members."[1] The tradition exerts a residual and unarticulated influence on the medical profession today. The tireless, dedicated physician struggling exhausted to his car after a 3 a.m. hospital call is scarcely aware of the influence of Hippocratic consciousness on his practice. Yet when efforts are made to challenge or revise the code, to modify it for recitation at commencement, reactions come to the surface, betraying unconscious emotive commitments born in the Hippocratic faith.

The code, as Edelstein, its leading interpreter, documents, is a reformed statement. It does not represent the consensus morality of Greek medicine but rather affirms a radical standard. It diametrically opposes the prevailing mores regarding infanticide, abortion, homosexual relations, the giving of poison, as well as the general health care ethos. The spirit of the Hippocratic Oath offers a fresh, humanistic, probably religiomystical alternative to the prevailing pagan ethos.

The Hippocratic ethical corpus embodied in the Oath, the Law, Decorum, Precepts, and other writings probably reflects a mystico-

Pythagorean religious anthropology and world view. Although the Asclepian[2] and Appollonian[3] elements are tacitly acknowledged, the deeper philosophic commitment of the tradition is Pythagorean.[4] The early Christians, still deeply influenced by the Hebrew views of life, saw the Hippocratic tradition of medicine as ethically noble and morally exemplary and sponsored its nurture in Western civilization. The tradition is therefore a product of Greek humanism claimed and perpetuated by the Christian Church into the development of the medical profession.

To survey the salient features of the tradition we must take a brief excursus through the history and then note the critical strengths and weaknesses in terms of contemporary relevance.

Initially we must see that the Hippocratic tradition is secular-humanist in its philosophic basis. Although there is a recognition of the Asclepian cult and certainly evidence of the mythicoascetic aspects of Pythagoreanism ("In purity and holiness I will guard my life and art"), the genius of the oath is that it anchors responsibility in the moral power and ability of man and does not concede to any transcendent moral law or moral arbiter. The evidence for the above interpretation stands in the (1) character of the developments in Greek natural philosophy stressing a demythologization regarding physical causality, (2) the ascendancy of rational-dialectical method in knowledge and the search for explanations, and (3) the prevailing influence of the Greek humanistic ideal of the good "healthy" person.

(1) The fifth century B.C. is the golden age of Greece, the Periclean age, the age of splendor. It is the age of the Milesian philosophers who probe the workings of nature and seek naturalistic explanations. Thales, Heraclitus, Pythagoras, and later Democritus, although all Greeks in that they see "the world full of gods," together seek the elementary explanation of natural movements, energy, flux, and process. Is it fire, water, air, or earth? Is there a fundamental atomistic constitution to reality? This broad philosophic tradition which investigated rather than accepted reality, which sought explanation without easy recourse to supernatural answers, is also the spirit of Hippocratic medicine.

(2) In Socrates a new epistemology is pioneered. Although the inductive and deductive methods remain strong and intensify in the Aristotelian and Platonic schools, the legacy of Socrates is to ask questions—to probe through the levels of evasive and nonrigorous explanation and to arrive at satisfactory truth which is at once objective and existential. In this spirit Hippocrates would not acknowledge epilepsy, "the Holy Disease," to be any more sacred than any other. Although the tradition later degenerated into sophistry and skepticism—asking questions for the sheer sake of questions—the essence of the dialectical epistemology is the quest for understanding in the service of self-knowledge and fellow-concern.

(3) Greek Olympian religion can be viewed as a search for the perfection in man. It is certainly an effort of anthropological idealization.[5] Greek athletics and medicine exalted the "ideal" person *kalosagathos*. The beautiful and the good went together. The glory of life is man himself. Man possessing the sound mind in a sound body *(mens sana in corpore sano)* is a god. It is this high humanism verging on godlikeness that is the glory and tragedy of both Hippocratic and modern medicine.[6]

The man-centeredness of this tradition mitigates against understandings which seek the normatively human from beyond man. When the Christians later affirm the intrinsic value of a deformed child, the anthropocentric value consciousness of the Greeks is contradicted. It takes a new consciousness based on *agape* for the weak, imperfect, and powerless to shape the Christianized Hippocratic tradition that controls Western medicine.

These elements of the search for natural as opposed to supernatural causality, the critical-dialectical method, and the emphasis on natural perfect man as normative constitute a cultural ethos which shapes Hippocratic medicine and with retrospective power exerts profound influence even today.

The strengths of the Hippocratic tradition are a vital center of responsible medicine today. The code emphasized the importance of covenant fidelity between the physician and pupil and physician and patient. Paul Ramsey in his Beecher lectures at Yale anchors this medical commitment in Hebrew-Christian theology which is the faith concept that propels the Hippocratic ideals into the modern world.

I hold with Karl Barth that covenant-fidelity is the inner meaning and purpose of our creation as human beings, while the whole of creation is the external basis and condition of the possibility of covenant. This means that the conscious acceptance of covenant responsibilities is the inner meaning of even the "natural" or systematic relations into which we are born and of the institutional relations or roles we enter by choice, while this fabric provides the external framework for human fulfillment in explicit covenants among men. The practice of medicine is one such covenant. Justice, fairness, righteousness, faithfulness, canons of loyalty, the sanctity of life, hesed, agape or charity are some of the names given to the moral quality of attitude and of action owed to all men by any man who steps into a covenant with another man—by any man who, so far as he is a religious man, explicitly acknowledges that we are a covenant people on a common pilgrimage.[7]

Today the idea of covenant responsibility has particular bearing in the area of social distribution of health services and the provision of medical care for all who require it. Medicine, as one of my medical students points out, is a social contract. Society has bargained with physicians to provide their education, to fund the basic research establishment perquisite to their art, to build the institutions necessary to their work. Now society asks the physician to activate his side of the covenant in a lifelong engagement to protect and maintain the health of the community that has called him into social covenant.

Erik Erikson in an address to a recent graduating class at Harvard Medical School stressed the necessity of interplay between covenant fidelity, rooted in the persons, and professions of medicine and the capacity to deliver effective care.

. . . fidelity is a virtue . . . meaning strength or inner force. It is a strength which must be firmly established before the next two stages of Love and Care can occur. . . . Identity and fidelity must precede Love and Care. It is because only a combination of identity, fidelity, and competence makes us able to be ethical.[8]

Fidelity is a touchstone of the Hippocratic tradition. Its recovery amid the highly institutionalized, specialized, technologized, anonymized activity that is modern biomedicine is absolutely crucial.

A second strength of Hippocratic wisdom in urgent need of recovery is its emphasis on a holistic-naturalistic conception of well-being. Listen to this advice from a fourth century B.C. physician:

> The cultivation of health begins with the moment a man wakes up. This should as a rule be when the food he ate the previous day has already moved from the stomach to the bowels. A young or middle-aged individual should take a walk of about 10 stadia just before sunrise, in summer however he should walk only 5, and older men will take a shorter walk in winter as well as in summer. After awakening one should not arise at once but should wait until the heaviness and torpor of sleep have gone. After arising one should rub one's neck and head thoroughly in order to overcome the stiffness caused by the pillow. Then rub the whole body with some oil. Those who are not accustomed to empty their bowels immediately after arising should perform this rubbing before the evacuation, while others will do it after evacuation but before undertaking anything else. . . . Thereafter one shall every day wash face and eyes with the hands using pure water. One shall rub the teeth inside and outside with the fingers using some fine peppermint powder and cleaning the teeth of remnants of food. One shall anoint nose and ears inside, preferably with well-perfumed oil. . . . The head is a part that requires a great deal of care, such as rubbing, unction, washing, combing, and close shaving. One shall rub and anoint the head every day but wash it and comb it only at intervals. . . . After such a morning toilet people who are obliged or choose to work will do so, but people of leisure will first take a walk. Long walks before meals evacuate the body, prepare it for receiving food, and give it more power for digesting it. Moderate and slow walks after meals mix foods, drinks, and gases contained in the body. . . . After the walk it is good to sit down and to attend to private affairs until the time arrives when one has to think of caring for the body. Young people and those who are accustomed to exercise or who need it should go to the gymnasium. For older and weaker people it is better to go to the bath or to some other warm place to be anointed. For people of that age if they have a gymnasium exclusively for their own use a moderate rubbing and light exercise are sufficient. . . . After such physical

exercise it is time for the mid-day meal, which in summer should consist of white barley groats with aromatic white wine well mixed with some honey and water—or some other gruel that does not produce flatulence, is nourishing and easy to digest. Those who do not care for such foods shall take cold bread. In addition to that, one shall eat some boiled vegetable such as gourds or cucumber, prepared simply. One shall drink white wine and water until the thirst is quenched, but before eating one should drink water in large quantity if one is thirsty, otherwise less. Soon after eating one should go to sleep in a shady or cool place well protected from wind. After the siesta one can attend to private affairs, take another walk, and go to the gymnasium. After exercising and being covered with dust, it is good for strong young people to have a cold bath. Older and weaker people, on the other hand, shall be anointed and rubbed gently and shall then have a hot bath. A general rule is that one should never or only rarely wash the head with hot water. . . . The chief meal is to be taken when the body is empty and does not contain any badly digested residue of food. Dinner should be taken in summer soon before sunset and consist of bread, vegetables, and barley cake. Dinner begins with raw vegetables with the exception of cucumber and horseradish, for these are vegetables that should be eaten toward the end of the meal. Boiled vegetables are eaten in the beginning of the meal. Other dishes are cooked fish and meats; kid or lamb meat shall be preferably from very young animals, pork from middle-aged pig, and as far as birds are concerned one shall eat chicken, partridge, or pigeon. All must be cooked simply. . . . Before dinner one shall drink water and continue to drink it some time afterwards. Lean people shall drink dark and thick wine and after the meal white wine. Fat people shall drink white wine all the time, and they all shall drink their wine with water. Fruits from trees are of little use, but if one takes them in moderate quantities before meals they do relatively little harm. . . . After dinner lean and flatulent people who do not digest well should go to sleep at once while others will take a short and slow walk before going to sleep. It is good for everyone to lie on the left side at first as long as the food is still in the region of the stomach, but when the abdomen has become soft one should turn to the right. It is not good for anybody to sleep on the back.[9]

Health involves the total activity of a person being in an environment. Socrates rhetorically asks Plato's Phaedrus, "Do you then think it possible to comprehend satisfactorily the nature of the soul apart from the nature of the whole *(tou holou)?*"[10] Biomedical ethics should be concerned with a total fabric of health maintenance, sustenance, and therapeutic care for persons. The genius of recent movements toward HMO's (Health Maintenance Organizations) where all the professions relevant to health are committed to providing a health-inducing milieu, though beset with political and professional entanglements, is a recollection of Hippocratic insight.

The weaknesses of the Hippocratic tradition deserve mention. The conceptions, medical and ethical, are pretechnological. The relevance of the tradition is limited when it comes to problems posed by the interposition of technology between health professionals and people.

The tradition focuses too much on crisis treatment as opposed to health maintenance. The model of the physician as a receptacle, to whom people come, certainly needs to be reexamined today. Finally, the very difficult questions of abortion and euthanasia, strictly disallowed in the oath, need to be reconsidered in the light of biomedical advances including at least genetic knowledge and amniocentesis, man-machine unification in the prolongation of life and the increasing appropriateness of electing one's time and manner of death. The tradition is rich and powerful. One who immerses himself in science comes to know he stands in the legacy of Greece. As one ponders the ethical substance of his private consciousness as well as that of his culture, again he knows that he is a Greek. To claim the great power of this tradition and retrospectively appropriate it into the ethical decision-making context today is a task of utmost importance.

# 2. The Religious Traditions: Jewish, Arabic, Catholic, Protestant, and Marxist

To distill the essence of the religious traditions that have shaped the modern biomedical ethos is a formidable task. We know the spiritual meaning of Moses, Mohammed, and Jesus. Perhaps we also know the medicoethical significance of Maimonides, Averroes, and St. Luke. Yet the cultural ethos in which modern biomedicine takes shape is only remotely conscious of the formative influence or lasting import of these religious traditions. For this reason it is appropriate to attempt to recover the original moral impulses that gave rise to the biomedical enterprise. This is done not to recapture for the now secularized professions and scientific activities some pristine goodness or restore some former religious hegemony. Rather the purpose is to initiate a genuine Socratic dialectic, a question and answer, regarding the relation of methods to ends—practical actions to purposes, immediate and ultimate—that the ethical quality of this most noble vocation might be sustained.

We are asking the religious traditions for what we will later call retrospective, introspective, and prospective insight. What light does the past have to shed? What are the present practical dynamics of interplay between the religious understandings of value (i.e., the sanctity of life, the natural goodness of procreativity, etc.) and the clinical arts of medicine? What meaning can the future bring?

In extremely broad strokes I now propose to paint the essential colors which constitute the health values of our main religious traditions. The Jewish, Arabic, Catholic, and Protestant traditions will be surveyed. These traditions are considered in their broad cultural power rather than in their restricted doctrinal content. Two reasons justify the inclusion of Marxism as a relevant religious tradition. First, it stands in the legacy of Judeo-Christianity and anticipates the modern faith of secular humanism. Secondly, one cannot miss the ethical fervor of Marxists at international conclaves on medical ethics.[1] This is such a fresh contrast to the relativistic skepticism of most European and American participants.

## JUDAISM

The faith of the people of the covenant and the promise has exerted a profound influence on the emergence of the modern biomedical ethos. Whitehead has shown how the Hebrew notion of time is basic to the whole scientific enterprise when joined to the Greek idea of the rationality of nature. The righteous energy of Yaweh in Jewish God-consciousness is surely the root of our quest for a better future, where pain ceases and peace reigns—that future symbolized in images of the Kingdom.[1]

The focus of this section is to take account of the fundamental Jewish faith and hope and *not* the meticulous moral tradition that is born in this consciousness. Jewish medical ethics are well summarized in two studies.[2] Judaism combines a deep, reflective ethical tradition with a detailed casuistry. Both elements are critical in assessing the tradition's moral view of health.

Salvation is the central motif of the Old Testament. God's history lifts up man's story into a blessed process whereby the creation is given with purposive quality and man is placed in the world as representative of God's dominion. The whole drama of nature and history is an activity of love and judgment, grace and forgiveness. Civilizations rise and fall; men respond and miss the mark; nature convulses and yearns for regeneration—all under the imprint of the redeeming Spirit of Yaweh.[3]

Man has an inalienable value because he is the creature of God. That is, a divine energy has given him the power to be; a divine image informs his nature and a divinely appointed purpose characterizes his destiny. One needs to live in the scientific world only a short time to understand how radical this anthropology is. It places an entirely different qualitative sense on the nature of man and therefore on the legitimacy of manipulations and transformations designed in modern medicine.

Man is given life in the divine Spirit. The soul *(Nephesh)* is breathed into man, sustained during biological existence, then withdrawn with the full incarnation of personality as the body expires and returns to the dust. Since each human life is a divine investiture summoned to responsible existence, man cannot do as he pleases with human being. Life is a gift, a stewardship to be responsibly exercised. When the Hebrew law sees the spilling of blood as "tantamount to expelling the divine presence from Israel," it reflects this noble estimate of man. There is, of course, no body-soul dualism in Hebrew thought as in Greek. The body bears a sacred significance. The laws against mutilation, personal injury, and burial illustrate this.[4]

In this basis of a divine imperative to love, a profound element in the medical ethos is born. The Jew is to love the stranger (Exodus 22:21); and recollecting Hebrew wisdom, the Christian is commended to have mercy on the enemy (Romans 12:14 ff.). The medical commitment to care for the prisoner; to serve the weak, defective, and advocateless; to guard the life of the unwanted and unproductive; is generated by this impulse.

It is this legacy that makes the modern medicoethical tradition so enigmatic. Neuremberg, the "Trial of the Doctors," and the resultant codes reflect on an epoch in which the value of life's intrinsic sanctity is turned upside down, and this in the body of Jewish humanity.

The abiding value of the Jewish anthropology is its localization of the moral imperative in the reality of God. Man is given not to value other persons because of utility or obligation but because God is God. The unconditioned character of the ethical impulse is a lasting value of the tradition.

Finally, man in Hebrew faith is a dynamic being, a person on the move. Just as Hebrew time-line injects a view of progress into history, Hebrew anthropology locates man's uniqueness in his possibility. Heschel says, "To animals the world is what it is; to man this is a world in the making, and being human means being on the way, striving, waiting, hoping."[5]

## ISLAM

Any account of the development of modern medical practice must deal with the critical role Arabic culture plays in the transition from the classic to contemporary world. In the eighth and ninth centuries Syriac-speaking Christians began to translate the classic works of Greek mathematics, medicine, and philosophy into Arabic. The recovery of this literature released a cultural renaissance that generated brilliant scientific and ethical insight. This contact with Greek ethics forced Arabic society to reject fully the sensual tribal values of the pre-Islamic period and develop the new precepts of belief and duty to Allah, forgiveness, moderation, charity, and kindness. The Muslim physicians, forced into ethical reflection with the recovery of Greek moral thought, forged a medical ethic that has endured into the modern world.

Since this tradition becomes the foundation of medical practice in the Renaissance and modern Europe, we mention its salient features:

(1) Al-Ruhāwis' treatise,[1] the principal document of ninth-century Muslim medical ethics, extols the dignity of the medical profession. Medicine is a profession given by God to those "whose hearts are pure, with a sharp intellect, and who love the good, have mercy, sympathy, and chastity."[2] The nobility of the profession is rooted in its commitment to sustain health, the deepest value of man. It is a priestly vocation, a ministry in the profoundest religious sense.

(2) The nature of this trust should prompt the most conscientious and delicate interaction with patients. The interview should be undertaken in tenderhearted manner; strict confidentiality should be observed. Intending the good should always eradicate any temptation to

do harm. These postulates of Islamic medicine, recollecting the gentle etiquette of Hippocrates, form the professional style of the modern physician.

The inclination of modern medical ethics toward etiquette can be traced to the Arabic recovery of Hippocratic ethics. The gentle wisdom of this plea for integrity between doctor and patient and the sanctity of his covenant is critical today. The privacy of covenant and passive-receptacle model of health provider of course needs drastic revision.

These insights come just in time. As modern medicine begins to probe causality in physical terms and therapy in technical terms, the necessity of this personalistic ethos is apparent. Interposed between the emergence of Judaism and Islam is the Christian faith, the world view and view of man to which we now turn.

ROMAN CATHOLICISM

The Associated Press recently carried a news item on the topic of sterilization. The case, originating in Missoula, Montana, concerned a young couple who had two difficult pregnancies, both requiring Caesarean section, one resulting in the death of the child. The woman was pregnant again. The couple had been denied sterilization operations because of Roman Catholic affiliation of the hospital. They were now bringing suit in federal court against the hospital. The case is built on the argument that the institution was the only public facility in a vast area that can perform this procedure. In addition, the hospital is supported by public money through state and federal programs and public fund drives. The hospital, the couple contends, should not impose its religious sanctions against persons of contrary commitment when it exists in this locale and under these conditions as a public institution.

The case raises the provocative issue of sacred and secular institutions and the maintenance of religious values in a pluralistic society. Of importance to our discussion is not the sociopolitical conflict but the bearing of a powerful tradition of medicomoral insight into the contemporary health ethos. Roman Catholic theology has generated the most thoroughgoing rigorous tradition of medical ethics that has ever appeared. The literature alone would fill a library. Of the many brilliant modern statements the work of Americans Kelly and Healy[1] deserve mention. Catholic theologians regularly address the issues and ecclesiastical positions abound. I scanned Karl Rahner's bibliography of some three thousand entries during a recent sabbatical and discovered over forty entries in medical ethics. The provocative encyclical *Humanae Vitae* is an example of the rigorous deliberations the Church brings to these issues. Our purpose in this brief section is to distill the genius of this tradition and assess its value in the contemporary situation.

In high level generalization Roman Catholic tradition stresses the goodness of the natural. John Noonan shows the way in which the Church historically formulates its objection to willful interruption of natural biological rhythms or developmental processes in its theology of procreativity, contraception, and abortion. Even the antinatural mood of Augustinianism, at least with reference to sexuality, is rationalized as a chastened naturalism. God has imbued human being with rich potential, having rational and physical dimensions. Total being fulfills its *natural* destiny only when sexuality is appropriately subordinated in the disciplined life.

Technical intervention is not only allowed but it is advised when the "natural" is facilitated. The following case from Healy illustrates this position:

Case 88
*Licitness of Olshausen and Gilliam Operations*
In order to correct the retrodisplacement of the uterus in a patient of childbearing age, Dr. X wishes to do an Olshausen or Gilliam Operation. The patient believes that the operation would be contrary to the Catholic code of ethics.
*Solution.* This operation is licit.
*Explanation.* The Olshausen operation and the Gilliam operation are in-

tended to relieve distress caused by the uterus and to facilitate childbearing. Hence there is no moral objection to this procedure. The patient misunderstands the purpose of the operation, and her fears should be set at rest.[2]

Not only is the "natural" normative in sexuality and procreativity, it governs in choice during life and death. The tension between ordinary and extraordinary means in a given medical context evidences the conscientious struggle to discern the natural (and by implication the good appropriate or obligatory) in a given situation.

The Roman Catholic moral tradition offers profound insight to the modern ethos. The tradition has weaknesses. The ethical heart of the tradition still needs to isolate historical colorations that compromise its relevance. Natural law ethics has been transmuted from its biblical possibility by stoicism, particularly in its propensity to fatality and resignation. The hierarchical jurisprudence of Roman law and the flesh-abnegating spirit of Neoplatonism and Augustinianism need also to be brought into proportion. A fresh reconsideration of Pauline understanding of law and Hebrew estimates of the body can help at this point.

The tradition has strong redeeming effect in our world so suspicious with the natural and so prone to the mechanical and technical. A recovery of natural law wisdom is one of the imperatives for philosophy, theology, and ethics today. In all of the problems of an advanced scientific world—ecological trauma, human manipulation, the technologization of life—the wisdom of natural law is urgently needed. We need to revere the rhythms, processes, and structures of nature. We need to see how man's creativity is at best a response to these orders, a utilization and amplification of them rather than a presumptuous distortion of them. Kepler noted that the grace to contemplate nature's wisdom preceded the ability both scientifically to discern and technically to utilize nature in a moral way.

The greatest challenge facing Catholic medical morals is to distinguish the unnatural from the natural as the latter is enriched by the range of human creativity. Is use of the prosthetic arm natural, ordinary means and therefore obligatory to consciences? What of the trunk prosthesis and the hemicorporectomy for cancer in the lower body? The fundamental question of qualitative human life forces this noble tradition to grapple with the profound ambiguities of modern biomedicine without the benefit of a black and white casuistry. The struggle of conscience and corporate ethical wisdom moves into the realm of ambivalence, mixed blessing, and curse as well as an at once heightened necessity to rely on rigorous exertion of reason and the grace of Holy Spirit. In this regard the tradition joins the ethical deliberations of Protestantism in facing modern biomedical crisis.

## PROTESTANTISM

To review the essence of Protestant moral thought to medical ethics is difficult because of the wide spectrum of contributions. Brilliant insights range from positions very close to Roman Catholic natural law viewpoints to innovative and nontraditional positions. My plan in this section will be to state what seems to be the distilled essence of Protestant morality, illustrating the view with the work of Paul Ramsey, Joseph Fletcher, and Helmut Thielicke. These theologians together with the now emerging work of James Gustafson[1] and André Dumas[2] are the major contemporary Protestant medicomoralists.

The unique insight of the Protestant faith is that of the radical graciousness of the divine acceptance of man and the resultant location of man's responsibility in the dimension of his freedom. Man is not condemned to any necessity, good or evil. His ultimate justification or salvation is not of his own doing. The ongoing demand for decision places on him the necessity to work out moral responsibility without the benefit of an elaborate casuistry or a natural law. He is under the demand of the moral imperative constantly, always aware of the ambivalence of good and evil in every option, always cognizant of the terrifying consequence of his decisions. He knows in faith that only grace can transform his act into a good. Even his noblest effort is ultimately tainted with self-interest. Ramsey, Fletcher, and Thie-licke work out the Protestant ethic with varying nuance. Each is responsive to this fundamental perspective. Though in concert they advocate the free realm of the conscience, each speaks differently of the way in which the conscience is informed and the way the ethical context should be understood.

Paul Ramsey[3] argues that life is covenantal by nature. Human beings exist in community in which the structures and dynamics of interaction have a moral quality. Covenant loyalty is at the heart of Christian ethics. God has initiated and sustained a gracious care of man in the covenant, and he calls on man to respond in similar manner. His act is indicative of what should occur in our actions.

God's covenant-creating-and-fulfilling performances . . . serve as the model for all performatives . . . from the nature of His self-involvement, men should display in their . . . covenants of life with life.[4]

The gift of life *(Gabe)* mandates the responsive task of care *(Aufgabe)*. Man is thrust into covenants by choice and into covenants which are not necessarily chosen. The medical covenant is one of the deepest and most sacred. It involves on the doctor's part the duty to heal, to save life, and to care with abiding constancy. The larger social contract which is the basis of health institutions and laws governing health are reflections of this basic covenant.

Love, the basic imperative of the covenant, demands of us responsible action, both in terms of deeds and rules. General and summary rules built up through history and the wide experience of cases enable us to exert a moral rigor in the analysis of ethical dilemmas in modern biomedicine. These rules seek expression in laws and professional codes. Codes of medical ethics render obligatory that which has been found to be normative in human experience. The view of the Church on abortion, widely compromised today except in Roman and Lutheran communions, according to Ramsey, is rooted in the covenant obligation to care for life. This care should not be abandoned in the name of any expediency. At the secular level the Neuremberg statute of informed consent is the humanistic extrapolate of the theological framework wherein common humanness entails that we recognize freedom in the person.

Ramsey's thought on cloning, abortion, organ transplantation, and euthanasia proceeds from this systematic foundation. He answers the fundamental questions, Why should I be just? or Why should I love my neighbor as a Jew? We love because God is God. There is no attempt to establish a moral imperative on utilitarian precept. But Ramsey does utilize the best thought of philosophical ethics. The unconditioned demand of Kant's categorical imperative is felt. The penetrating wisdom of John Rawls' notion of the original position and justice as fairness is implicit. The strength of Ramsey's contribution is found in the way he roots moral dynamics in a theologically understood creation. The insights of Ramsey are difficult to translate into immediate decisions because of a lack of detailed casuistry and because we still await his discussion of the dynamics of human decisions. Our subsequent discussion of a synthetic decision-making model attempts to appropriate his thought into this frame of reference.

If Paul Ramsey can be said to represent the pole of Protestant thought demanding the rigorously informed conscience, Joseph Fletcher pleads for conscience that ranges free in response to concrete cases still strongly guided by the love imperative. Fletcher argues that the classic modes of doing ethical analysis (i.e., legalistic and intuitive) are not adequate to the profound moral crises that are carried by technology. The extreme of a code morality always does injustice to the dynamics of concrete situations, and the extreme of antinomianism degenerates into an expediency ethic. Arguing that regard for persons and response to love commandment imply "situation ethics," he pioneers a model of decision-making that has great appeal to clinicians, if not to philosophers.[5]

The greatest good in any situation is maximizing the presence of agape, person serving love.[6] This value becomes axiomatic in the sense that it is the only inviolable principle in a decision-making context. Prefabricated regulations of a legal or religious character violate the dynamic quality of a given crisis because they seek to lift the timely into the realm of the timeless.

A family crisis with which I have been involved illustrates this problem. Mrs. X is a forty-six-year-old woman who has von Reckling-hausen's disease, a rare disorder that affects the central nervous system and causes multiple tumors to develop in the brain and elsewhere in the body. She has had twenty operations on her brain and is now in irreversible coma. Before she became comatose eight months ago, she signed a document developed by Fletcher and others called "the Living Will." This document, distributed by the Euthanasia Society of America, asks that physicians and hospitals not take active steps to prolong one's life in the case of incurable, terminal illness.

Mrs. X was for several years before the onslaught of the disease an intensive care nurse. She knew firsthand the inhumanities of prolonged illness on patient as well as on family. The mother and father witnessed the signing of this document. When it was presented to the attending neurosurgeon, he claimed he could not heed its directives, however humane, because of several inviolable rules. He was obligated as a physician to preserve life and not abandon care (which adherence to her wish would entail). He was subject to a hospital guideline which required continued feeding of persons in irreversible coma, and he feared the ever-present possibility of *ex post facto* litigation by the parents. At last check the patient still lingered. The parents were ridden with guilt for not having insisted on their daughter's wish, thus compounding the life-altering burden of care and financial obligation. The doctor and all others attending the patient were deeply cognizant that in this case ethical commitments to life might indeed be inhumane.

Fletcher would argue that the impulse of agape, disinterested love, would prompt the pragmatic and utilitarian response of positive intervention to end the life of Mrs. X. Her personal intention would be served. The correlative command of doing no harm, though immediately violated, would in the long run be served and the total humanity of the situation would be served.

Fletcher's ethical schema has enlivened the discussion of specific clinical cases. It has positively responded to Daniel Callahan's critique of traditional ethics wherein there is no response to concrete dilemmas:

If I may put the matter in the form of a paradox, the ethicist may be quite correct in his theoretical analysis—perhaps utilitarianism is, say, the largest philosophical issue at stake in many ethical dilemmas. Yet he will be quite clearly wrong if he does not recognize that the issue in particular cases—Mrs. Jones in Ward 5 at 4:10 in the afternoon—must and will involve far more than the status of utilitarian theory.[7]

Our best philosophical and theological theorists have not made application of their thought to these areas because the disciplines have not been able to make the transition into a modern anthropology where human being is seen in its dynamic quality and the ethical context itself is understood as ongoing process. This challenge to contextual relevance has been the lasting contribution of Fletcher.

The weakness of his thought, of course, is the weakness born in the immaturity of the art of medical ethics. A rapidly developing biomedical technology day to day renders yesterday's "good uncouth." Acceptance of death in leukemia children, just yesterday a noble value, today is an irresponsible resignation. Remissions are frequent and the traditional wisdom of accepting boundaries would constitute a failure to care. Yet the emphasis on the ethical context as an ever-fluid setting distorts the living reality within which men's lives take place. The time-established values of the Neuremberg codes illustrate this. Even though specific, immediate experiences (the testing of a new chemotherapeutic agent in cancer on a dying child) might require suspension of the stipulation of long animal trials, the stipulation itself has enduring value. A "shooting from the gut" ethic now characterizes medicine. It undergirds the impatience of doctors with endless philosophizing which never makes up its mind. It is evidenced in the chafing experienced under drug laws and human experimentation guidelines by physicians. Yet this enduring wisdom has been established at great cost and deserves to be perpetuated.

The ultimate danger of Fletcher's position is that it abandons radically the belief in the normatively human. A recent essay on "Criteria for Personhood"[8] toys with the frightening proposal that the humanum is nonexistent and that ad hoc criteria—timely and situational, always modifiable as science advances—should guide us as we seek to serve and preserve human being.

At this point the work of a modern German medical ethicist helps us. The anthropotheological constrictions of Dietrich Bonhoeffer[9] and Karl Barth[10] set the stage. Helmut Thielicke's work constitutes the most extensive Protestant treatment of modern biomedical problems.[11] His reformulation of the concept of "borderline" situations *(Grenzsituationen)* retains biblical profundity and philosophical consistency in relation to highly ambivalent modern problems. In this regard he solves the problem of Ramsey's scholasticism and Fletcher's relativism.

Thielicke contends that life is structurally ordered according to the divine purpose. Human existence is constituted in man's creation. The orders of creation and fall *(Schöpfungsordnungen, Notordnungen)* inform nature and man's life with meaning. Co-humanity *(Mitmenschlichkeit)* and being for one another constitute the purpose of man's sexuality and his broader family and social status. But man's being in the world *(in-der-Welt-sein)* is not utopian or nostalgically or pietistically otherworldly. He exists in concrete history with all the uncertainty, ambiguity, and mystery that life brings. As he lives in faith and responsibility in the midst of crisis, he grows into maturity.

Man is aware that his disturbed existence is but a reflection of the profound disorder that marks his relation to others, to world, and to God himself. In the meantime he lives under the mark of the fall, always aware that alienation characterizes his existence and malice or hubris his actions. Since the fundamental relatedness of his life is to God exhibited through his life with the neighbor, he experiences his behavior and decisions under judgment and grace. In this theological ontology man's being and act are related so that one cannot view the value of a person either in some pure essence alone or in terms of function. Man has an indelible dignity because he is the chosen creature, fashioned in God's own image. His dignity does not attest to some intrinsic goodness; rather it is bestowed on him in grace. His preciousness is given by God as dignity (virtue) is given him *(fremde Würde)*.

The problem of abortion or the interruption of pregnancy (tubal ligation) represents a borderline situation. It is borderline in two senses. It occurs at the boundary of one of nature's spheres of existence (sexuality and marriage). In this sense it intensifies the ambivalence of a given decision because of the way a given decision seems to enhance or enrich the fundamental order (the well-being of a family) even when the act is destructive of life. Borderline situations also clarify the essential nature of the good structure of existence (love, in this case), since they are such "propitious places for acquiring knowledge."[12] In pregnancy the arm of God has been extended to man; his gift has been proffered. The noble status of parenthood, motherhood, and fatherhood has already been given. Therefore, any abortion for social, economic, or convenience reasons is unjustifiable. Society should structure itself in ways to accommodate life thus brought into the world when the child is unwanted.

The presence of medical indications and therapeutic abortions reveals the full complexity of the borderline. The new technologies of amniocentesis (endoamnioscopy, sonar testing) and abortion allow a wide range of fetal aberrations to be known. Should a Thalidomide child with multiple defects be brought into the world? What of a Tay-Sachs child? Now the case presents itself of the possibility of testing for Huntington's disease.[13] Surely the entree into the human community of grossly distorted and even mildly "abnormal" represents an evidence that we live "between the aeons." Is our responsibility to bear with outrage the affront or to launch a vigorous program to "wipe out" birth defects?

Thielicke would argue that it is our responsibility to obey the love command in creation with its correlate not to kill (murder can be expressed in wish and thought). Yet we need to proceed urgently with medical knowledge to diagnose illness, to develop therapeutic measures (insulin for diabetes), and always to be prepared to bear the consequences of intervening actions. For example, we have sought to obliterate malaria, one of the distortions of nature consequential of the fall, by widespread hygienic and public health measures. We have created in this action a massive burden of hunger, starvation, and overpopulation. We need to bear the consequences of this intervention as a global community by economic and technological measures which are alone appropriate.

The Protestant stance on medical ethics can be summarized as a strong affirmation of human responsibility activated in the free realm of one's conscience. This conscience is informed by the eternal ordering of nature disclosed in the Word; by the responsive interactions of persons, whereby God's will is known in the needful plea of the other; and by the eschatological vision, wherein man is called not only to wait but to persevere with patience (acceptance of boundaries) after the coming Kingdom where "death shall be no more, neither shall there be mourning nor crying nor pain any more, for the former things have passed away" (Revelation 21:4, RSV).

The sociopolitical ethic is at once activistic in the reformed traditions and quietistic in the Lutheran and Methodist traditions. The former faith calls under judgment the sociopolitical structures which dehumanize man. The latter serves as a constant warning against the utopian fallacy. Both traditions have a strong legacy into the contemporary biomedical ethos.

### MARXISM

A brief comment is in order with reference to Marxist medical ethics. The concern is intense in the Soviet Union and eastern Europe. Medical students in the Soviet Union must take nearly 400 hours in Marxist-Leninism. At worst the course is political indoctrination. At best it is very sophisticated thought on medical ethics.

The social ethic is most strongly emphasized. There is a personal professional code which has some affinities to Hippocratic and more personalistic Western counterparts. The great emphasis, however, is laid on the physician's obligations to society. He is a servant of the growth of the human community. He is to serve the health of his nation and undergo whatever sacrifice this entails. He will very likely be sent to the rural villages upon completion of his training, and he is expected to serve for the normal remuneration given to public servants. His code puts a stress on preventative medicine, health maintenance, and, of course, crisis care. The clinics that are situated with an enviable distribution around the country serve the people of that vicinity. The scruples against abortion and euthanasia are certainly not so intense and fraught with emotion as they are in America. Yet the visitor senses a profound reverence for life in the Soviet Union. Perhaps this is the legacy of a deeply religious people and the passion of Russian Orthodoxy. Perhaps it is the new areligious humanism of Marxism wherein man becomes the ultimate value.

I have mentioned earlier the deep imprint made by Latin American Marxists at a recent scientific meeting in Mexico City. Perhaps a great step toward the formation of a global humanity and a more humanistic quality in a mechanized world can be achieved by discussion and cooperation with Marxist brothers. The Christian-Marxist dialogue in Europe is a beginning in this direction. Holding even greater promise is the scientific and biomedical interchange now beginning. We can hope that Eastern and Western bioethicists will soon meet together for exchange. Perhaps in this way a fire of humanism, perhaps even a spiritually charged[1] commitment to man, can be forged to counter the insidious process of technologization of man now compromising all human value.

# 3. The Neuremberg Tradition

William L. Shirer, historian of *The Rise and Fall of the Third Reich*, begins his discussion of "The Medical Experiments" with these words:

There were some practices of the Germans during the short-lived New Order that resulted from sheer sadism rather than a lust for mass murder. Perhaps to a psychiatrist there is a difference between the two lusts though the end result of the first differed from the second only in the scale of death.

The Nazi medical experiments are an example of this sadism, for in the use of concentration camp inmates and prisoners of war as human guinea pigs very little, if any, benefit to science was achieved. It is a tale of horror of which the German medical profession cannot be proud. Although the "experiments" were conducted by fewer than two hundred murderous quacks— albeit some of them held eminent posts in the medical world—their criminal work was known to thousands of leading physicians of the Reich, not a single one of whom, so far as the record shows, ever uttered the slightest public protest.[1]

Shirer adds the note:

Not even Germany's most famous surgeon, Dr. Ferdinand Sauerbruch, though he eventually became an anti-Nazi and conspired with the resistance. Sauerbruch sat through a lecture at the Berlin Military Medical Academy in May of 1943 given by two of the most notorious of the doctor-killers, Karl Gebhardt and Fritz Fischer, on the subject of gas gangrene experiments on prisoners. Sauerbruch's only argument on this occasion was that surgery was better than sulfanilamide! Gebhardt was sentenced to death at the so-called "Doctors-Trial" and hanged on June 2, 1948. Dr. Fischer was given life imprisonment.[2]

The ethos of modern medicine, particularly in its experimental aspects, is profoundly shaped by the tradition of Neuremberg. In this section we will first survey the gruesome historical circumstance that precipitated the "Trial of the Doctors." Then analysis will be made of the formulation of the code of ethics and the central insights of this tradition. Finally, a critical evaluation of the code will be attempted.

One can now walk across the open fields where not long ago stood the transit stations, barracks, and experimental labs of the Dachau internment camp. In the summer of 1972 Jewish leaders from around the world visited the ignominious sight, driving the short distance from Olympia Stadion in Munich where a tragedy would soon break recalling that horror now thirty years past.

Traditions began in the nineteenth century which brought German culture and medicine in particular to its vulnerable point. The beginning of fraternities, the insidious beginnings of anti-Semitism, the ethnic pride, are all there in the late 1800s. Several developments, frighteningly similar to developments in the United States today, began to occur. Medicine began to be pressured into the public domain. The physician was no longer an individual entrepreneur. He was responsible to express the values of the social order. The fundamental Hippocratic commitments were gradually compromised as the physician-scientist became a technician. Nineteenth-century German medicine, it should be recalled, was unexcelled in the world. Medical students around the globe had to know the German language to enter the realm of biomedical literature and research.

The state became involved in promoting health insurance, and the profession was seen to have a greater and greater social function. The emphasis on preventative medicine and public health led in the 1920s to eugenic measures in which the overt desire was to perfect the Nordic species by eliminating defects and impurities. It is easy to see how noble values, values we again pursue in contemporary medicine, are so easily distorted.

The medical crimes of the National Socialist government sprung in part from these eugenic values which justified sterilization, the least of the inhumanities inflicted on the Jews. Other values serving military purposes also prompted many experiments. Prisoners were placed in pressure chambers and forced to endure high altitude atmospheres until they died. They were guinea pigs to test the effects of weightlessness and rapid fall to simulate the effects of a high altitude airplane accident. They were subjected to freezing experiments in ice and snow.

Even more heinous were the crimes labled K tenology (the science of killing) by Ivy and others. Prisoners were injected with lethal doses of typhus and jaundice. They were given gas, gangrene wounds, bone grafting, direct injections of potassium and cyanide into the heart. They were dissected alive to watch heart and brain action. At the macabre height of the experiments the only motive was to collect different shapes of skulls and retrieve skin to make lampshades.

How could it happen? In a Christian society, in a society possessing the unexcelled cultural brilliance that could nurture a Bach, Beethoven, or Brahms? Dr. Andrew Ivy, A.M.A. representative at the Neuremberg trials, commented:

The ethics of medicine were violated by the Nazi physicians (and, through silence which amounted to complicity, by a large part of the German medical profession). . . . No it appears to me that this "Witches Sabbath" of medical crimes was only the logical end result of the mythology of racial inequality and of the gradual, but finally complete encroachment on the ethics and freedom of medicine by the Nazis when they were in the process of gaining control of the German government. And this process . . . went unopposed by the German medical profession.

As a result the world witnessed the catastrophe of a national medical group which let itself be ruled by a false political ideology and found a notable number of its members committing murder under the defense of political expediency and superior orders.

Had the profession taken a strong stand against the mass killing of sick Germans before the war, it is conceivable that the entire idea and technique of death factories for genocide would not have materialized. From all the evidence available, it is necessary to conclude that far from opposing the Nazi State militantly, part of the German medical profession cooperated consciously and even willingly, while the remainder acquiesced in silence.[3]

## The Neuremberg Code:

1. The voluntary consent of the human subject is absolutely essential. This means that the person involved should have legal capacity to give consent; should be so situated as to be able to exercise free power of choice, without the intervention of any element of force, fraud, deceit, duress, overreaching, or other ulterior form of constraint or coercion; and should have sufficient knowledge and comprehension of the elements of the subject matter involved as to enable him to make an understanding and enlightened decision. The latter element requires that before the acceptance of an affirmative decision by the experimental subject there should be made known to him the nature, duration, and purpose of the experiment; the method and means by which it is to be conducted; all inconveniences and hazards reasonably to be expected; and the effects upon his health or person which may possibly come from his participation in the experiments. The duty and responsibility for ascertaining the quality of the consent rests upon each individual who initiates, directs or engages in the experiment. It is a personal duty and responsibility which may not be delegated to another with impunity.

2. The experiment should be such as to yield fruitful results for the good of society, unprocurable by other methods or means of study, and not random and unnecessary in nature.

3. The experiment should be so designed and based on the results of animal experimentation and a knowledge of the natural history of the disease or other problem under study that the anticipated results (will) justify the performance of the experiment.

4. The experiment should be so conducted as to avoid all unnecessary physical and mental suffering and injury.

5. No experiment should be conducted where there is an *a priori* reason to believe that death or disabling injury will occur; except, perhaps, in those

experiments where the experimental physicians also serve as subjects.

6. The degree of risk to be taken should never exceed that determined by the humanitarian importance of the problem to be solved by the experiment.

7. Proper preparations should be made and adequate facilities provided to protect the experimental subject against even remote possibilities of injury, disability, or death.

8. The experiment should be conducted only by scientifically qualified persons. The highest degree of skill and care should be required through all stages of the experiment of those who conduct or engage in the experiment.

9. During the course of the experiment the human subject should be at liberty to bring the experiment to an end if he has reached the physical or mental state where continuation of the experiment seems to him to be impossible.

10. During the course of the experiment the scientist in charge must be prepared to terminate the experiment at any stage, if he has probable cause to believe, in the exercise of the good faith, superior skill and careful judgment required of him, that a continuation of the experiment is likely to result in injury, disability, or death to the experimental subject.

Of the ten principles which have been enumerated our judicial concern, of course, is with those requirements which are purely legal in nature—or which at least are so clearly related to matters legal that they assist us in determining criminal culpability and punishment. To go beyond that point would lead us into a field that would be beyond our sphere of competence. However, the point need not be labored. We find from the evidence that in the medical experiments which have been proved, these ten principles were much more frequently honored in their breach than in their observance. Many of the concentration camp inmates who were the victims of these atrocities were citizens of countries other than the German Reich. They were non-German nationals, including Jews and "asocial persons," both prisoners of war and civilians, who had been imprisoned and forced to submit to these tortures and barbarities without so much as a semblance of trial. In every single instance appearing in the record, subjects were used who did not consent to the experiments; indeed, as to some of the experiments, it is not even contended by the defendants that the subjects occupied the status of volunteers. In no case was the experimental subject at liberty of his own free choice to withdraw from any experiment. In many cases experiments were performed by unqualified persons; were conducted at random for no adequate scientific reason and under revolting physical conditions. All of the experiments were conducted with unnecessary suffering and injury and but very little, if any, precautions, were taken to protect or safeguard the human subjects from the possibilities of injury, disability, or death. In every one of the experiments the subjects experienced extreme pain or torture, and in most of them they suffered permanent injury, mutilation, or death, either as a direct result of the experiments or because of lack of adequate follow-up care.

Obviously all of these experiments involving brutalities, tortures, disabling injury, and death were performed in complete disregard of international conventions, the laws and customs of war, the general principles of criminal law as derived from the criminal laws of all civilized nations, and Control Council Law No. 10. Manifestly human experiments under such conditions are contrary to "the principles of the law of nations as they result from the usages established among civilized peoples, from the laws of humanity, and from the dictates of public conscience."

The value insights from the Nueremberg experience will long endure. They provide vivid directives to current activity involving research in human subjects. Probably the greatest contribution is the sharpness it brings to the criterion of informed consent. All of the code's stipulates revolve around this point. The scientific value must never become an end in itself. It must always be directed toward the subjects, and if scientific interest results in human suffering disproportionate to the benefit, it should be discontinued. The modern clinical practice of attempting full disclosure of risk, side effects, and potential harm is a dimension of this value. The right to terminate the trial or one's involvement in it at any time is affirmed. The criterion needs to be followed most rigidly when dealing with experimental populations prone to passivity and abuse. The subjects should understand fully the implications of the trial and communicate back to the investigator their understanding. When prisoners, minority groups, children, the mentally retarded, medical students, or any other "special" group is selected, the stipulates should be followed with meticulous care.

There is great value also in the code's attempt to evoke a humanitarian ethos. The trials and resultant documents search for "laws of humanity," "dictates of public conscience" on which norms of human decency can be established. In a secularized civilization where a plurality of values interplay, it is critical that we search for this constellation of basic morals. This should not be a reduction to "street morality." Worse yet, we cannot settle for a "least common denominator" of shallow "eclectic" ethic. The easy solution of relativistic ethics can be overcome if we probe deeply into the nature of man, his perceptions of the good, his resistances to manipulations, and build an ethic upon this "common sense."

Anthropologists now see the inadequacy of earlier models wherein values were seen to be radically culturally determined and nonobjective. With the insights of Claude Lévi-Strauss, Margaret Mead, and others, we can now see the basic structure of human personality and the valuing capacity common to all men. Lawrence Kohlberg has noted stages of moral development[4] which are cross-culturally unanimous and predictable. A universally acceptable moral framework— nonreligious, although it may be derivate of theological tradition; nonsectarian, although it should express the depth of particular moral traditions—is vitally needed today. It is imperative as a condition for meaningful world law, world government, and global science policy.

The most important ethical insight from Neuremberg is the reminder it gives to the potential evil in man. Even in this high culture, advanced in rationality and science, this barbarism can occur. The experience serves as a constant refutation of the myth of inevitable progress. It shows the levels to which a civilization sinks under technologically influenced totalitarianism and mass hysteria. Objectification of man into disease entities and pathological specimens, the process necessary to sound scientific medicine, is also its potential downfall. Objectification can easily lead to manipulation and ultimately lead to abuse and sadism. The Neuremberg experience reaffirmed the locus of a human society to be in the informed conscience subject in the final analysis not to custom or law but to the moral law alone.

The weaknesses of the code have been highlighted by Beecher.[5] The criterion of informed consent is never fully applicable. Consent is simply "not there for the asking" (Beecher). Most trials and experiments have implications unknown even to the investigator. Even if the known 450 counterindications of a given drug were known, they could not be communicated in a meaningful way (presented, then reiterated by subject to show comprehension). Even computer and teaching machine mechanisms of *informing* the subject will never prove completely satisfying of this criterion. We are cast back on the fundamental human virtues of trust and honesty: genuine concern for the other. The code is a guideline. Like a red traffic light, it influences behavior. Yet the Neuremberg code, fully accepted and implemented, will never substitute for the conscientious person. Human research should continue, guided by the rigorous standards of Neuremberg and related codes developed by institutions and associations. The constraints should not be seen as impediments to a flourishing experimental medicine, but rather as signposts that direct such research to the service of genuine human needs with means commensurate with human values.

# PART TWO

---

## A Model for Decision-making

---

# 4. Sources of Ethical Insight

**Sources of Ethical Insight**

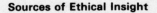

Memory
Retrospective
Insight

The decision-making context

Hope, Prediction
Anticipation
Prespective
Insight

Awareness, Love
Introspective
Insight

Although it is important to understand the context within which a given decision takes place and the traditions which have sustained values, it is yet another task to discern the present sources of ethical insight. The good does not always emerge obviously or self-evidently from the raw experience. I will argue in this section that insight for decision-making and planning comes from three directions. Indeed the traditions of ethics we have analyzed are sensitive to these three vectors. The Hippocratic tradition has highlighted the way that value is built in, constitutive of reality. The religious traditions have accented the dynamics of responsiveness to a present source of goodness. The Neuremberg tradition is built on the ethics of consequences. Just as modern theology recognizes the juxtapositional wisdom of memory and hope converging to enlighten the present, so medical ethics can discern value from the threefold direction of human perception. Man's memory allows him to appropriate the "what has been" with meaning. Love and awareness allow him to be responsive in the present. Hope and prediction allow him to read the future.

First, there is retrospective insight. This value proceeds from history. The estimate of man that undergirds this value rests on a view of his endowment or his nature by creation. Philosophically, we are here concerned with the natural rights of man. HUMANITY is a generalized concept that underlies the value we place on particular human individuals. Classic philosophy called this the *humanum*. Ethical understandings of man from this perspective can be biologically controlled and determined. This view might contend that man's inherent worth resides in his vitality. It can also be philosophically conceived. From this perspective man's reason, with the correlates of freedom and responsibility, form the basis of human value. In the Greek philosophical and religious mind human life has value because of its eternal character and its purposive quality, its nature and destiny. All of these perspectives on man with their implicit norms come to bear on the processes of decision-making and planning. An anthropology and ethic, affirming what man is, what he can be, and therefore what can be done with or to him, is carried in these perspectives. These sources of insight are borne into the decision-making context by the humanistic traditions and histories, philosophical and religious.

Secondly, there is introspective insight into the good in a given situation. This value flows from the present living reality of man's being in the world. Here values are dynamic because they are rooted in the act and being of particular persons at particular times in particular circumstances. Here we deal with the phenomena of conscience and common sense. Here we face the feelings of guilt and satisfaction, the vitalities of love and denial, the willing of the good and the destructive. If norms for decision-making and planning flow from the meaning of human life in retrospective insight, they flow from the dynamic present processes of life in the introspective insight.

Thirdly, there is the source of ethical insight which might be termed prospective. Here we deal not only with meaning and being, the history and present of man, but also with his possibility and future. Here also we concern ourselves with his technological extensions. Here insight proceeds from the future, from that which is possible. Here we deal with the proleptic question of what man might be. Here we are concerned with consequential insight. What will be the consequences of this or that particular action? As far as the human actor is concerned, we must evaluate the possible results, the side effects, and the response that might follow a particular action. As far as the technology itself is concerned, it must be prescriptively determined what the impact will be on the person and what the feedback cycle will throw as return signal. The norms that proceed from this direction are, of course, probabilities. It should be noted, however, that technical predictabilities are much more certain than human predictabilities.

In summary, sources of ethical insight can come from behind, within, and ahead; from memory, from the depths of being, from beyond; from the past, present, and future. Responsible decision-making and planning should be aware of these three vectors impinging on any particular decision-making context. Let us now examine these three sources in detail and example.

(A) The imprint of the past etches itself on the moral consciousness of man in a variety of ways. Tradition affirms what man is by nature. Jewish faith, for example, holds that man is a creature. This means that his life is conditioned by, and contingent upon, his Creator. Values that flow from this anthropology include strictures against self-sufficiency and idolatry. When a human being fails to acknowledge that the source and power of his being is rooted in God, or when he locates trust in self or some penultimate reality, he violates his humanity. The implication of this value for biological life is that human vitality is a stewardship, and a possession only in that sense. Conversely, this value would warn against man setting himself up as arbiter over life and death. When man seeks to become Lord over the coming and going of life, he usurps the prerogatives of his creator, shatters the creature-creator relation, and ceases to be a man.

A wide range of mandates flows from this kind of traditional value to those situations where man's life is coupled with a mechanism or empowered with a technology. Many of these situations, of course, impinge on life and death. Many ethical dilemmas present in the new technology can be resolved through memory and wisdom in the light of this tradition.

Human values which are thus rooted in historical consciousness are generally codified or otherwise perpetuated in legal and religiomoral traditions. Sometimes these are affirmed as divinely established norms, sometimes as self-evident axioms. Sometimes the values are affirmed as human insights and constructions, learned through experience and therefore verifiable at the practical level. One generation appropriates this value to the next through education, communal religious life, and personal influence.

A good example of retrospective value insight comes in the area of human experimentation. The Neuremberg statutes, which inform so much of the current discussion on medical ethics, also have power in their historicity. They say as it were, "This you have learned—never let it happen again!" One cannot comprehend the caution and concern that pervades situations of clinical experimentation today apart from the influence of the Neuremberg history. In nations closer to the history—Germany and the Soviet Union, for example—the consciousness is heightened. Witness the reluctance to heart transplantation in those countries. America and the rest of the world pay great respect in clinical experimentation to the Neuremberg principles of thorough animal testing, informed consent, and precedent of patient's interest over the scientific value.

(B) The present *"Sitz-im-Leben"* (life situation) with its dynamic qualities of choice is becoming a forceful perspective on ethical decision-making today. In this understanding the moral question is not so much "What is right?" as "What is best?" The "now" context of value formation is very skeptical of metaphysical or absolutistic norms. In the existentialist mood the perspective often contends that values are subjectively created; they do not objectively exist. Fortunately, we are now becoming wary of this mischievous dichotomy. The good must have objective reference if it is to have subjective power. But also it must live in human action if it is to have reality. The way in which ethical activity is rooted in personal psychic and social behavior is a great contribution of the behavioral sciences to the moral quest.

Common sense and conscience become receptive instruments of this source of ethical insight. The moral agent in touch with "common sense" level of feeling can often filter out the good from the morass of expediency, social pressure, and psychic hangup factors that so often obscure the decision-making situation. "What makes sense—for me now and all others concerned?"

Immanuel Kant argues that a good will in a person presents itself to our common sense as intrinsically good. It is not justified by any utility. The good will (encompassing action in Kant's sense) is a total intentionality within which the good is recognized and pursued. It is not contingent on reason or on consequences. It has validity in and of itself.[1] The immense value of Kant's legacy in modern moral philosophy is to rescue ethics from the crass expediency of utilitarianism, the obtuse formalism of rationalistic theorists, and the unpredictability of intuitionism. The brilliance of these traditions synthesized with the genius of utilitarianism is brought to the modern discussion by the work of John Rawls.[2]

Rawls seeks to integrate the principle of utility which presents itself in a compelling manner to human reason with the subtler moral sentiments of man. Rawls does this by a reconstruction of the social contract theory of obligation in a Kantian mode.

The heart of the Theory of Justice born in this tradition is "the original position." The fundamental association that forms a community and precedes any social contract occurs when the initial position of equality is affirmed. Basic rights and duties proceed from this understanding as fairness becomes the norm of interactions. Inequalities or injustices are tolerated only if they benefit all. "Inequalities of wealth and authority are just only if they result in compensating benefits for everyone, and in particular for the least advantaged members of the society."[3] Far from evoking a utilitarian standard at this point (poverty is justified if social good follows as consequence), Rawls is recovering a biblical value, implicit in the moral philosophy of Kant, wherein "the least of these" (the weak, the retarded, the advocateless, the sick, the aged, the child, the fetus) is placed in a unique normative position. His good must be affirmed for justice to exist.

One of my outstanding students, Michael Hemphill, has shown in an unpublished paper the relevance of this theory for the ethical dilemmas created in the new genetics. He argues that sensitivity to the values of justice in social interactions will prompt us to special responsibility to those whose life we would biotechnically alter. We must put ourselves in their position, or better, transpose all parties vested with interest to that hypothetical, original position where the imperatives of justice as fairness become clear. The "golden rule" invoked at this point is invested with Christian meaning wherein the good wish for the other is not simply enlightened self-interest (even in the noble sense of Kant's universalization principle) but a genuine commitment to the well-being of the other even to the point of self-sacrifice.

The value of reading situational interactions in this introspective way is found simply in the fact that willing the good of the other makes "good sense." When this introspective insight, enriched as it is with utilitarian and intuitive insight, is further deepened with retrospective and prospective value insight, a helpful model of the decision-making context is found.

Although most often harmonious with common sense, conscience sometimes gives overriding counsel. Without going into the theological subtleties of the nature of conscience, it operates as an instrument which perceives the good—despite, over against, even in contradiction to what we feel or think—or what makes sense. I feel that conscience is the "extra sense" that anchors man in wisdom to the greater meaning and purpose that human life is and has beyond its immediacy. Although the psychodynamic distortion that conscience can be put to is clear, history is replete with the examples of supernatural perception and vision that it can mediate into man's active life of decision.

This introspective dimension of ethical insight is actively operative in the area of abortion today. At the level of personal dynamic and public policy, we see the terrible tension between common sense and conscience. Common sense prompts us to respond sympathetically to women in desperate need and make clinically sterile, legal and economically feasible abortion available on request. Conscientious concern for the sanctity of fetal life and social affirmation of the value of life prompt a contrary action. Although this concern will be raised in the illustrative section on generating man, the power and limitation of the introspective source of ethical insight must be noted at this point.

If memory and faith (in its confidence quality) are the psychic contacts with the retrospective source of insight, awareness and love are the introspective contacts. Much less clear, more ambiguous, yet more powerful and demanding are these perceptions. Awareness is earth-shaking in its revelation, love-compelling in its demand. H. Richard Niebuhr argues very simply that ethical maturity is a responding awareness to "what is going on."

(C) The future is the most baffling, yet most critical direction from which our ethical insight must come today. I had to create a neologism for this insight: *prospective.* The dominance of this category in the current discussion is at once hope-engendering and frightening. We are obsessive about the future in America. We live progressively. We contort and distort the present in the "forward-looking" compulsiveness that is our engrained Puritan heritage. Nevertheless, the magnitude of the problems demands of us this painful reading of, and responsiveness to, the future. Wolfhart Pannenberg writes:

Within the present human reality ethics must discover the tendencies toward the possible amelioration of present life. Honestly confronting what is, ethics must point to what is to be, what can be, what ought to be.[4]

In the area of technology and man's life we are dealing with the proclivities of hope and planning, anticipation and control. Contemporary man claims more and more control over the unknown and the "yet to come." Both Marxist and Western Christian thought speak of man's "becomingness" (*Noch-Nicht-Sein:* Ernst Bloch). Does man wait for his future or does he create it? How can the "not yet" be a source of ethical insight? As we ponder these questions, we see the impact of technology. Technology is a tool to create the new, to make the future. Because of control and communication (the feedback mechanism) more aspects of human life are claimed from the realm of chance and programmed with predictability.

The future sends ethical signals in two ways. First, there is the insight that comes from man's hope to be something, his possibility. What man can become is now a very powerful determinant of what he decides to do. Secondly, there is the signal of consequence. Technology gives us the capacity to predict or foresee the consequences of certain decisions. This new fact will have staggering ethical import in the next decades.

One of the most powerful zones of convergence of theology and science today is the element of the future. If God is the power of the future (Moltmann), and man is the creator of the future, new theological definitions of co-creativity and responsibility are needed.

The ecology problem will illustrate this point. In the grand scale enterprise of man's utilization of natural resources through his mechanical intervention into the natural environmental processes, he creates devastating feedback, mainly because he does not know what will happen if he does something. He usually crosses his fingers and hopes. DDT immediately reduces the incidence of malaria. What follows, who knows? Today we can begin to see the future's handwriting on our wall. We are beginning to see what interventions do, not only to hydro-, atmos-, and biospheres, but to man himself. If we can begin to perceive the challenge of the good and the undesirability of the bad from the future, great ethical advance will be ours.

This brief excursus on sources of ethical insight has been studied and highly abstract. Yet it is a necessary backdrop to my approach. It now needs the fleshing out of specific problems. I choose a range of human situations where a technology is joined to human life to create a new ethical context. In each the reader will note the presence of promise and threat, of good and evil. In each he will find a resolution—a normative statement—a suggested direction to go. I have tried to avoid the vocational hazard of ethicists, resorting to questions when practical dilemmas arise, never declaring one's mind. Many times in straining for the prophetic, the thought becomes apocalyptic and alarmist. This reflects the commitment that the moral is living and active, not abstract. Many times discussion of the problems will become sermonic. No apology is made for either passion. This only reveals the way I personally tremble in the face of these challenges and the way I yearn for that new day when the only impositions on life fulfillment for each human being will be self-chosen.

# PART THREE

---

## Modern Designs and Transformations

---

# 5. Generating Man

The most fundamental way that modern man seeks to apply technical skill to his own life is through genetic alteration and reproductive biology. A wide range of practical considerations ranging from amniocentesis and abortion to technical transformations of childbearing, extrauterine gestation, etc. fall within the spectrum of activity I will call generating man. Genetic ethics is a field that combines acute personal and family crisis with a profound futuristic implication for the human race. Several case studies that have concerned our Institute exemplify the present day-by-day dilemmas created in this new biotechnology.

Mr. Sam Brown is a twenty-two-year-old black married male. He is a graduate student in one of Houston's law schools. His wife, a university graduate, is now preparing to enter medical school. While skiing last year in Colorado he suffered an attack of abdominal pain and severe weakness while at the top of a mountain. Following a preliminary diagnosis of anemia, he was returned to the care of his Houston physician. Further tests disclosed that he had sickle-cell anemia.

The condition was brought under immediate medical management and the couple sought out consultation on the attendant problems of life adjustment. At our Institute we have an interdisciplinary team composed of internists, geneticists, psychiatrists, and pastoral counselors. Numerous new challenges faced the young family. Should Sam continue law studies with the view to a political career even though his life expectancy is drastically shortened? Could his wife continue her medical education? Would it be impossible and/or unwise to have a child?

In addition to supporting the family our team weighs the broad cultural questions and seeks public policy action at local and national level. Why has so little money been invested researching this disease so common to our black populace? What would be the positive and negative aspects of genetic screening? If mass testing revealed, as some predict, that 10%–15% of the black population carry the trait, what kind of family guidance would be humane both for present individuals and potential offspring?[1] What of the genetic load consequences?

The maturity and religious faith of this couple is enabling them to cope effectively with this severe blow. The disease is under management. Some hope is afforded by new methods of chemotherapy. The couple is following with great vigor their original career plans; in fact, they now claim fuller joy from each moment and each experience. They have been compelled by circumstances to ask the ultimate questions of meaning and destiny. They have seen the challenge of weighing profound values. Like other families we see, the Browns teach us the wisdom of appropriating the insight of the past, sensitively understanding the dynamics of the present, and discerning the future.

The case of Mrs. Levy came to our attention when physicians in Buffalo, New York, asked for a consultation. The family, possessed of high religious scruples, had had one child with Tay-Sachs disease. This degenerative disorder of the central nervous system produces severe retardation and early death. When Mrs. Levy accidentally became pregnant, she went for amniocentesis and other tests to determine the genetic profile of the fetus. Several tests gave what appeared to be conclusive evidence that the child had the disease. After much contemplation and consultation, the family decided on abortion. The abortus was completely normal. The shocked family had been cautioned regarding the inconclusiveness of the tests used. Still they had not been prepared for this result. From traditional faith they affirmed the sanctity of life and decided on abortion only with great hesitation. With the exception of the diagnostic data which was highly convincing, the situational evidence was varied. Family and friends counseled both immediate abortion and allowing the pregnancy to go to term, hoping against the evidence for a normal child. The consequential considerations weighed strongly against having another affected child. The case vividly points up the limitations of genetic knowledge and technology. It highlights the deep conflict of values that accompanies decisions in the area. It points to the awesome weight of bearing the consequences of decisions made.

The futuristic-social dimensions of generating man can be seen in two instances of public concern. In New Jersey a family with a hemophilic child is suing the state for costs of care because it did not make available to them preventative knowledge. I am told by a reliable scholar that a major private health insurance is contemplating the policy of requiring amniocentesis or other acceptable forms of antenatal diagnosis for all pregnant women holding policy with the company. If a diagnosis of congenital defect is made, insurance will be dropped on the potential child. In other words, abortion will be required. Metpath, Inc. of New Jersey is now offering the service of cytogenetic analysis called "banding" to physicians around the country. The chromosomal studies from blood cultures promise to "aid doctors in determining the risks potential parents face in producing children with mental, physical and behavioral deficiencies."[2]

In this chapter we will survey the background of scientific and technical development that brings us to our present state of genetic knowledge. We shall then determine the basic anthropological questions inherent in this knowledge and technology. Attempt will then be made to search the pathways of traditional, common-sense, and predictive insight that might render normative values into these crises. In conclusion, specific guidelines will be suggested derivative of this understanding of man.

The ultimate ethical issue of genetic knowledge is that of creating life and remaking man. Genetic modifications are but intermediate expressions of this ultimate capacity of generating and replicating life. Cloning, therefore, becomes an "ultimate consequence" kind of case that must be considered side by side the immediate practical dilemmas. Indeed, one of the troublesome implications of recent cancer biology is that knowledge to create life may have to precede knowledge to correct genetic distortion. Robert Sinsheimer of Cal Tech has pointed to the fact that genetic engineering, amniocentesis, and abortion may be only stopgap necessities until we can perfect in vitro fertilization and gestation, tetraparental and perhaps interspecies chimeras—fundamental alterations that will make phenotypic and genotypic therapy unnecessary.[3]

Our knowledge in biology is rapidly giving us this capacity to do a wonderful and frightening thing: to create life from nonlife, to fabricate man. The process began in a Munich brewery in the late 1800s. A brewery chemist working with that good Malz decided to test the vitalism concept of Pasteur which claimed that vital process could occur only within the living cell. Büchner homogenized living yeast cells, added sugar, and produced alcohol. For the first time vital biochemical process occurs outside the sacristy of the living cells, and man knows it.

The momentum accelerates into our century. Muller notes the homeostatic dynamics of genetic breakage and rearrangement in the thirties. Beadle ushers in the age of molecular biology in the forties. Avery and his colleagues discover the dynamics of cell synthesis in the nitrogen processes involved with nucleic acids: DNA, RNA. Then in the fifties Zamennic and his Harvard colleagues synthesize proteins for the first time outside a living cell. The sixties bring Kornberg and Lederberg, the synthesizing of DNA with the full genetic activity of natural DNA. Then at the turn of the decade Beckwith and his colleagues isolate and photograph the gene. In recent years attempts to fabricate the gene promise the logical outcome to this chain of events. Knowledge becomes power; facility to know becomes ability to create.

Technology develops parallel to this genetic knowledge. The tools become sophisticated and the clinical capacities enlarge. Petrucci in Bologna follows the differentiation of a human embryo for sixty days. Human life, previously nurtured only in utero, is sustained in vitro. The artificial uterus and placenta begin their entree as mechanical counterparts of those natural functions. Drs. Edwards and Steptoe of Cambridge successfully implant a laboratory fertilized egg in the womb of a London woman. At the more practical level, amniocentesis coupled with the growing acceptance of abortion for genetic as well as medical indications greatly enhances our ability to determine what kind of person will be born.

Our present technologies are frightening in their power, and they are only the beginning. They are frightening for one simple reason: they enlarge our responsibility. We will soon have the anticipatory knowledge, and therefore the responsibility, of choosing the kind of beings we allow to enter the human community. Our present technologies are several. There are the techniques of preconception screening such as the tests for Tay-Sachs propensity and sickle-cell anemia. There is the technique of diagnosing sloughed-off fetal cells in the amniotic fluid with amniocentesis. Dr. Carlo Valenti in the recent issue of the *American Journal of Obstetrics and Gynecology* introduces the amnioscope which with very low risk can obtain tissue biopsy and blood sample from the fetus.[4] Future instrumentation will very likely render primitive these tools we now have to discern the kind of human being on the way toward birth.

The prophets of doom have their day as do the writers of science fiction and the pious moralists. Albert Rosenfeld announces the Second Genesis.[5] *Esquire* announces the second Noahic covenant saving earthly life from extinction after the ecological apocalypse.[6] A single Easter bunny is launched to some planet or platform in outer space. Her uterus is implanted with the germ of every animal species: two elephants, two hippopotami, all in a clean and sterile prenatal environ, refreshingly sweet-smelling, at least when compared with Cecil B. DeMille's ark.

And so it goes. The fall of man is seen in its full biblical ambivalence. It is both fortunate and tragic. It lifts him to an unsurpassed height of science and pre-science. It takes him to the brink of hell. He gains mastery over inexorable mystery. He becomes the maker and giver of life. He is summoned to "come and play God." "We are not sure," in the words of Robert Sinsheimer, "whether we face an ambush or epic opportunity."[7] We ask in our excitement and terror, "Shall we make and remake man? Shall we tamper with the building blocks of life? Shall we play God?" Perhaps we decided affirmatively long ago when as Prometheus or Pandora we first controlled fire or took a drug. Man decided to play God when he first sought to alter natural process. We do it again and again when we treat a wound or build a dike or receive an inoculation. Today, although the question is given profound dimension, we are asking an old question: "Should man play God?"

Does the creativity of man conflict against, coexist alongside, or cooperate with the divine creativity? Is man's emerging skill in genetic control a usurpation of divine prerogatives, a thinking his thoughts after him, or has man at long last taken hold of his responsibility of co-creativity in cosmic subjugation? Has God yielded this power to man who is finally come of age?

We are dealing in these areas with a profound exertion of man's dominion over life. The ethical issues in the genetic manipulation of man can be gathered around the theological themes of *creativity* and *procreativity*. Here, of course, we are dealing with the biblical mandates to "fill the earth and subdue it" (creativity), and "be fruitful and multiply" (procreativity) (Genesis 1:28, RSV). Responsibility thus anchored in transcendence necessitates the belief that man is placed on the earth to keep life wholesome, to protect it from assault, and to transform life according to his finest vision of humankind's future. The ethical directives proceed retrospectively, introspectively, and prespectively from these theological motifs.

*Creativity:*

In considering the issue of creativity we immediately confront what appears to be the major issue in this sphere. It is expressed in Paul Ramsey's question, "Shall we clone a man?"[8] or Shamai Kanter's question, "If man creates life, is he still man?"[9]

Man has achieved great creative sophistication in his evolutionary advance. Chemistry and the cognate technologies recreated and initiated process in that field. Agronomy and agriculture brought control and novelty into plant life. Domestication and breeding gave man new discernment and manipulative skills with animal life. Now the secrets of human life begin to reveal themselves. The normative question presses in forcefully. Should man seek to reduplicate human life? Shall we clone a man? How should we manipulate the germinal determinants of human life?

Although we now accept evolution as the scientific truth about man's emergence, establishing the transbiologic uniqueness of man, the *humanum,* is a more difficult matter. Faith contends that the qualitative uniqueness of man is not naturalistically derived but born retrospectively into our history and transcendentally into our ethical consciousness.

This estimate of man is portrayed in the strange, paradoxical anthropology of the Bible. "What is man?" cries the Psalmist. "Thou hast made him little less than God, and dost crown him with glory and honor" (Psalm 8, RSV) Jesus asks, "Look at the birds of the air. . . . Are you not of more value than they?" (Matthew 6:26, RSV).

The Bible talks to us symbolically and therefore forthrightly. Man is dust. He is clay from which the potter shapes a vessel. The pot does not rise up and question its maker. The Lord can smash it in pieces like a potter's vessel. From *"ādāma,"* from mud, earth: man, Adam, is fashioned and the breath of God gives him life.

Man becomes a living being *(Nephesh Adam).* Into his nostrils rushes the breath of God, the Spirit *(Ruach Elohim).* The same wind that activates the primeval waters, animates man. "We have this treasure . . . in earthen vessels" (Genesis 2:7; Psalm 2:9; Isaiah 64:8; John 1; Romans 9:21; II Corinthians 4:7). Man alone is made in the image of God, or as the Bible prefers to talk about it, man is empowered in his breast with the breath of God. Theologically, this is linked to the Spirit of God—the Healing, Holy Spirit.

What are the genetic implications of this synopsis of biblical anthropology? Let me venture this: it is not the flesh and bones, not the genes and chromosomes, not even the great heart or sophisticated brain that makes man something valuable, not the stuff of man, the matter and the mechanics. It is his spirit—given in creation; sustained in the few short years of biological life; called forth in one's being with others; captured in the eternal, redemptive will of the Creator. The spirit of man—call it personality, or soul, call it moral being—is not identical with, or detached from, any physiologic function. It is not in the heart or kidneys or brain. It informs and is informed by man's total being: biologic, psychic, sociorelational.

So how does our question look in the light of this sketch of the Bible's description of man? Shall we clone a man? Can man clone a man? We can keep a few cells viable in cold storage in Bethesda. Perhaps we will create tissue cultures. Perhaps we can build cellular aggregates that will perform organic function. But can we make a man —a man with a soul? Soul, with all that it means: lineage, historicity, destiny, transcendent reference! Perhaps soul is something man is given, not something he has. Ian Barbour argues that man should welcome the power to create life and not quickly flee its challenge.[10] I would prefer to argue that theological ethics mandate man not principally to create life but to protect and enhance the life we have been given. How paradoxical that we should aspire to fabricate man when we so neglect the developmental possibilities of existing persons!

In the more immediate challenges of genetic engineering, genetic surgery, positive and negative eugenics—what prerogatives should we take in terms of transforming human life? If we shrink from the ultimate ethical legitimacy of giving and taking life, what are the intermediate consequences? Are we justified in bringing diabetics to childbearing age through insulin therapy? Are we responsible for the public maintenance of sickle-cell anemics or invalids with congenital kidney disorders requiring hemodialysis? What are our positive and negative, our creative and protective responsibilities?

The scientific progress that has brought us to this point is at once thrilling and terrifying. One can only feel that the profound insight is given as a challenge to enlarged responsibility. A thought that staggers the imagination is the way that macrocosmic reality is microcosmically present. The universe whirls in every living cell. How awesome to realize that all the information for the organism exists in each single healthy cell. This realization staggers our minds because it seems to be a deliberate, willful disclosure to us by God of a profound mystery. It is as if the Lord entices human investigation and imaginative creativity by disclosing profound mystery in utter simplicity. It is as if he says, "Come and see, and know, and use; but be careful how you use."

It should be clearly evident that I am arguing for an understanding of human creativity which sees it as mutuality with divine creativity. I prefer to think of human ingenuity as co-creativity with God.

Most practical problems rest on the dilemma of how we use our knowledge. Corrective genetic engineering involving phenotype and perhaps even genotype may be justified to release a person to full life. Negative eugenics raises few questions except those of feedback and increased genetic load in the race. We think of congenital malformations, mental retardation, cancer, diabetes, PKU, Hemochromatosis, galactosemia, Wilson's disease. Who could deny that the unlocking of these secrets, the discernment of techniques of genetic alteration to effect cures, avoiding the necessity of the interim tragedy of abortion, would be a great good. It might not be an unqualified good, but a great good—worthy of man's energetic striving. Otherwise, we believe in some demon god who wills disease, destruction, and debilitation. There is no disagreement on this point. Surely we are meant to transform human life toward its designed wholeness and potential.

But what of positive eugenics? What of novelty creativity as opposed to corrective alteration? Shall we clone a man? Whose man shall we clone? Who says who will clone whom? Some serious scientists still argue the genetic deficiency of the black and the poor. Shall we refine the race? Who is your model "*Ubermensch*"?[11] When creativity becomes captive to demonic purpose, which military purpose always is and political purpose most frequently is, then we contradict the moral purpose of reality and invite destruction.

What kinds of genetic proposals are we dealing with? Herman Muller calls for a deep freeze sperm bank.[12] We keep the sperm of superior man; check this out after a twenty-year lag, then proliferate the progeny of men who prove to be virile, sensitive, compassionate, etc.

The French biologist Jean Rostand and the American Nobel Prize winner, Joshua Lederberg, argue for genetic engineering that will enhance and enlarge the mental abilities of man to cope with the technological future he has created.[13] Weitzel of Tübingen calls for a worldwide genetic campaign to abolish all diseases to "create a world with less suffering."

It would appear that the immediate ethical challenges are going to arise with the joining of amniocentesis and abortion techniques. As we gain sophistication in antenatal diagnosis, a wider range of abnormalities will disclose their presence. We will be able to detect a wide range of metabolic disorders, the presence of various congenital diseases affecting the central nervous system, many forms of mental retardation. We can now determine the sex of potential children. We may one day be able to determine the propensity of a nascent person to cancer and cardiovascular disease. The burden of the knowledge will be significant. We may concur with Bentley Glass in his stipulation that all children have the right to be born normal.

We may agree with Marjorie Shaw, one of the world's outstanding geneticists who works in our center in Houston. She argues that genetic disease is the same as communicable disease, albeit vertical and not horizontal in transmission, and therefore should be isolated and quarantined as a public health measure—not allowed to transmit itself. She argues that we have the legal obligation to protect the unborn from "the cruel and unusual punishment" of genetic disease.[14]

Surely we need to ponder whether the abnormal merit our protection, even in utero, and what deviation from the *norm* is abnormal. New knowledge and technology intensify our responsibility. We now have the possibility, which means responsibility, of deciding whom we will admit to the human community.

Most challenges of ethical decision-making in genetics are not the broad speculative questions, but the crisis of day-to-day choices. Should we risk having a defective child since we are both carriers of a defective gene? Should I, as a physician, tell the whole truth and thus discourage a family into complete resignation? What should our posture as society be toward the retarded, the handicapped? What levels of persuasion and coercion are permitted in guarding the strength of the gene pool?

In all these proposals we need to walk the thin line between titanic aspiration and acquiescence. Man should not become so enamored with his power or the might of his hand (Deuteronomy 8:17, RSV) that he feels that the biological future of man depends on his taking hold of the evolutionary process and shaping it to his intentions.[15] On the other hand, he must not lapse into some powerless withdrawal where he sees his creative efforts to be futile in the light of some inexorable process. In other words, man must not allow himself to choose the easy escapes of genetic apocalypticism or the apathetic acquiescence that shrinks from the enormity of the problem.

A theological understanding of creativity in this profound dimension of genetic life would call for an attitude of awe and humility. Man should stand silently and reverently before the glorious and terrifying possibilities of that future that his creativity will fashion. Hopefully, his activities of scientific perception, technological implementation, and feedback anticipation will be colored by the hues of mystery and awe. Perhaps we can call this prespective intuition. Hopefully, the objects of his research and technique will be seen as objects of value and meaning. It is only this attitude that can discern the good and the true. "Only when the spirit hath learned to contemplate [betrachten] what God hath made," says Johann Kepler in his wisdom, "will it learn also to do what God hath commanded." Only as one is deeply, ethically absorbed in the profound meanings of what he is doing, can he operate creatively or co-creatively.

In summary I am suggesting initially that the creative impulse given man is symbolized in the biblical mandate to "fill the earth and subdue it." Two theological understandings serve meaningfully to direct genetic creativity. They provide ethical insight retrospectively to these decision-making situations. The first is an awareness of biblical anthropology, which sees man as personal-spiritual being in creation and destiny. The second is an operational attitude of reverence and ethically controlled perception in genetic research and manipulation.

### Procreativity:

The practical ethical decisions in this area usually concern human procreativity and the inalienable value of personality. Here we hold as backdrop the biblical summons "be fruitful and multiply." Muller's proposal of semen banks; the implications of the work of Petrucci and others researching (in vitro) embryo nurture; the whole range of "programmed prenativity" that Albert Rosenfeld speaks of, raise the basic issue of the normative understanding of human sexuality, love, and procreativity. Here we shift to an introspective level of ethical insight.

Again the illustrative problem of cloning sharpens the ultimate question of genetic knowledge and engineering. The genetic issues that concern us here are several. What are we doing when we conceive life apart from the love consummation of man and woman? What are the implications of developing human life in a contrived artificial environment substituted for the woman's body? What kind of breach of natural process is involved when a genotype is fashioned that has no precedents? Does life make any sense if it is radically discontinuous from any stem? Is nonemergent, nonhistoric being meaningful in any sense? It is like the man conceived by artificial insemination who every Father's Day sent a box of cigars to a syringe in Denver, Colorado. After John Kennedy was assassinated, this question arose among those of a Frankenstinian bent, some friends of mine in fact. "If we were only advanced enough to take a yet viable cell from this dying man and decode and differentiate that information, we could make a new JFK as life lapses in the original." Does that kind of ahistorical life make any sense? At what point do our genetic alterations fulfill human life and where do they violate a wisdom of nature necessary to mankind's future?

In addition to these issues which focus on the identity of man we must also consider the great socioenvironmental questions that have a genetic aspect. Here the press of the future has prespective ethical import. Should the genetic material be manipulated to avoid a global population catastrophe? This might mean selective sterilization based on socioeconomic or intelligence factors. It might mean the withholding of corrective genetic manipulation in certain negative eugenic situations, deciding not to counter the natural selection process with our scientific ingenuity. Let natural selection and survival of the fittest do its thing. It could mean some form of genocide for the sake of survival.

These concerns throw us back to the biblical anthropology in its procreative aspect. The Lord says, "Be fruitful and multiply." How are we to understand this mandate in an age when population control and not proliferation is the moral imperative? Let me propose some insights from what might be called a theology of procreativity.

Considerable variance exists, of course, between Roman Catholic, Jewish, and Protestant theologies at this point. We have noted how Roman Catholic thought seeks to interpret in a fresh and relevant way theological imperatives that protect natural sexuality, conception, and nurture.[16] We should guard the private conscience and cherish the cultural wisdom enshrined in this tradition.

Jewish theologies stress the awesome responsibility of the procreative life and the imperative to marry and propagate the race. "To refuse to do so," says the code, "is tantamount to bloodshed and to expelling the Divine Presence from Israel."[17] The tender sensitivity of a Mrs. Levy, the familial commitments, the willingness to sacrifice for the community, are integral components of our "winnowed wisdom."

Protestant theologies, as usual, afford a smorgasbord of thought. Paul Ramsey speaks of the covenant context of procreative responsibility: ". . . in human procreativity out of the depths of human sexual love is prefigured God's own act of creation out of the profound mystery of his love revealed in Christ."[18] Helmut Thielicke calls attention to the polarity of sexuality, the erotic determinants of man's biological nature, and the way in which sexuality and procreativity constitute fundamental expressions of this basic order of life. Human life fulfills earthly destiny and prefigures eternal destiny as sexual love is fulfilled in the birth and growth of children. Eros and Agape interpenetrate in this profoundly holy, human activity.[19]

William Pollard, the scientist-theologian, compelled by the environmental crisis, reasons somewhat differently as he takes issue with the "yesterday, today, and forever" anthropologies:

. . . in the remaining third of this century man will have fulfilled the biblical injunction to be fruitful and multiply and fill the earth. But an inescapable corollary of this injunction faces us now with terrible urgency. Because the earth is in fact a spaceship for man's journey, it is essential that once the earth has been filled by man, he must *stop* being fruitful and cease further multiplication. Moreover, this must be accomplished within a generation, or certainly within no more than two generations. The children of today's college graduates must, as they approach adulthood, already have started the process which their children must complete; namely that of separating human sexuality from procreation.[20]

Paul Ramsey counters by pleading that there be no "complete or radical 'in principle' separation between the personally unitive (love) and the procreative aspects of human sexual life."[21]

The theologicoethical imperative which emerges from the procreative mandate can be seen in a resolution of the tension between Pollard and Ramsey. The introspective and prespective values are not in real conflict on this issue. Ethical responsiveness must hold the creative and procreative impulses together. The biblical injunctions of creativity and procreativity are joined, counterbalancing imperatives. These impulses are given man as complementary gifts. They are to enhance each other. Man is meant both to guard life and to transform it. When procreativity threatens creativity, it must sublimate so that abundant human life can ensue. How are the two mandates linked?

First, it must be noted that man is created in a global family. Von Rad carefully notes in his exegesis of the passage (Genesis 1:26–28) that God's creativity controls the passage (*bara*); that *mankind* (*ādāma*, plural) is created, not *man*. Luther instinctively translated this correctly: *Menschen*.[22]

Secondly, the passage emphasizes that "thouness" is fundamental to man. There is no male and female. Man is designated for the "thou" of the other sex. There is no man, only man and woman.

Finally, and most important, Von Rad notes that procreation is not related to *Imago Dei*—to God's image in man—but rather to *blessing*.

This seems to mean several things. It clearly indicates that human sexuality and procreativity are instrumental to God's glory. Man is bound to world community in being and destiny; he is not an island. Responsibility means that he is bound responsively to organic world community. Finally, man's procreativity is given in covenant blessing (with the responsible reciprocity that entails), rather than in his divinely constituted nature. In short, sexuality is to be used conditionally, not unconditionally.

Pierre Teilhard de Chardin speaks of both the cosmic communality and sublime futuristic aspects of procreativity.

... love is tending, in its fully hominized form, to fulfill a much larger function than the mere call to reproduction. Between man and woman, a specific and reciprocal power of sensitization and spiritual fertilization seems in truth to be still slumbering, demanding to be released in an irresistible upsurge toward everything which is truth and beauty.[23]

To me this indicates that man is responsible for his use of life and the creation of a future. This is what genetic science is all about. Genetic ethics requires the rich insight from all directions of our decision-making model. Genetic manipulation is a terrifying capacity full of ambivalence. It is a technology full of threat and promise. It is a capacity of science and prescience without which man cannot survive.

The following case illumines this problem area and the way our model of decision-making may be used. Mrs. X came into the genetics center at our medical school with the following request. She was twelve weeks pregnant and wanted amniocentesis to see if the fetus she carried was male or female. Together with her husband, she had made a decision that they wanted only one child and it should be a boy. The presenting reasons were many, most having very little force other than personal taste. A son could inherit the family goods. He would perpetuate the family name. He could fulfill athletic ambitions missed by the father. The geneticist-physician faced a twofold dilemma. On the one hand, should he perform the amniocentesis? On the other hand, could he conscientiously perform the abortion if the fetus were a female? There was a burden of responsibility in administering the test and sharing the knowledge. Certainly the action of abortion was fraught with ethical significance.

The physician elicited several consulting opinions including my own. He weighed carefully the retrospective insight. The value of life: the Hippocratic commitment to do no harm by inducing abortion became vivid and demanding. The responsibility to protect vulnerable life from assault—female life at that—recalled the deep Judeo-Christian value of compassion to the weak and advocateless.

At the introspective level he had to understand the terribly ambivalent dynamics. Certainly he had the responsibility to care for his patient, the mother. The husband and wife had some tension on the issue. The father apparently desired the male child more than the wife. Sharpness of conscience in the couple was blunted because of various pragmatic and convenience issues. In addition to these there were the interactional signals from medical colleagues, medical school policies, and community awareness.

From the prespective insight a powerful signal emerged regarding the ethical use of this new technology. The basic wisdom of nature's sex ratio was questioned. Universalizing the action, and in this sense pretesting the consequences of a particular action, provided a conclusive answer for this physician.

He decided against both the test and the abortion, but provided reference to another center where the desired services were available. In a sense this was an evasion of duty. In a deeper sense it was a compromise based on the profound ambivalence of the situation and his fundamental respect for the private conscience of his patient. He would not function as technician and merely carry out her desires. On the other hand, he affirmed the personal prerogatives of his patient. The woman would have perceived the ethical context differently, her husband in yet another way. The various relevant others—family, lawyer, spiritual adviser—also sensed the moral dynamics differently. All perspectives contributed to a holistic frame of reference within which professional and patient ultimately bore the burden of decision.

Conception control and abortion become the options for the time being in response to our scientific knowledge and ethical signals in determining the entrée of potential or nascent human life into the world. This means we must bear the consequences of *allowing* or *not allowing* human beings to be born. At this point of history responsibility would seem to be great if we choose to bring new humanity into the world. Although the hysteria over population explosion was overstated, particularly in the United States, the mandate is still clear. We must plan *care*fully for the persons we bring into the world and we must pre*pare* the world for them in order that they be wanted and their life be wholesome.

Margaret Mead notes:

I think that one should place abortion first within the context, that we are free today at least to discuss the possibility of not giving birth this week to every little human soul beating against the window of life.[24]

Mead argues that a humane ethic thinks more about the living than about the unborn. Today this clearly means restricting potential life, and perhaps in some instances nascent life, for the sake of the quality of life for earth's present family. These after all are the persons for whom we are now responsible, and we are not doing a very good job. A negative intervention, a playing God, if you will, seems imperative, but the action has its consequences. Dag Hammarskjöld sets the terror of this responsibility in his *Markings.*

If you fail, it is God, thanks to your having betrayed Him, who will fail mankind. You fancy you can be responsible *to* God: can you carry the responsibility *for* God?[25]

Now the other side of the coin: in the section on creativity I argued that the essential meaning of operating on God's behalf is that man not aspire to be God, but recognize ultimately his boundary, his finitude. Ethics in this case is the acceptance of the hope compromised by the boundary of the possible. Responsibility today requires man to "play God," but not aspire to be God. Some elaboration of this latter danger seems important right now. The postulate of the sanctity of human life has as a correlative, the human right to life. This means social and political decision to protect human life, to preserve its freedom. In the abortion arena today this means preserving a human being from assault. Sometimes a person must be protected from the physician and medicine. Sometimes a person must be protected from his lawyer and the law. Sometimes a person must be protected from his priest and the church. Sometimes a person must be protected from himself. These are the parameters of radical freedom. These principles are imperfectly implemented in modern political orders. They are radically asserted in Jewish-Christian anthropology.

The retrospective insight of biblical theology shows that the assertion of life or death control over another person is to set one's self up as God. In Hebrew thought idolatry is to contort God into man's image or coerce God's will to man's. In the Old Testament, Life is given by God. It is the breath of God that activates man. "Thou fashioned me in my mother's womb," cries the Psalmist (139:13). Job perceives that the Lord gives and takes away and He is blessed (1:21). In Christian insight Jesus is the author of life (Acts 3:15).

What does a full-orbed ethical analysis suggest for clinical decisions and public policy regarding abortion? Let me list several convictions in conclusion.

(1) A humane society should not only allow but facilitate abortion when a mother's well-being, a family's vitality, is severely threatened. It should be readily available and economically feasible. The woman who has conceived a new life in love, and then undergone the agonizing crisis of deciding to terminate that life for medical, genetic, psychiatric, or sociologic indications, has paid the moral price. Society should not constrain her from "playing God." In this sense the 1973 Supreme Court decision which affirms the precious covenant of physician and woman patient as ultimate arbiter is sound and humane.

(2) The physician, who will become the principal counselor in abortion situations, should not hide behind the wall of not "playing God", nor too readily jump in and "play God." He should clarify the medical and psychological indications, help locate the decision in the realm of personal responsibility, and stand by his patient in support, strengthening her integrity and responsibility.

(3) In public policy we must press for completely safe preventative birth control techniques. We must clearly state that it will not be public policy to consider abortion an option in the armory of birth control measures. We certainly cannot conscientiously accept a future like the present where abortion is the most widely practiced form of birth control in the world.[26] We must state that when nascent life is thus dehumanized, a whole range of human value affirmation is cast aside.

(4) The law should protect personal freedom and the integrity of doctor-patient relationship. This would imply an absence of coercive

law prohibiting or condoning abortion. We now need to broaden public policy in order to encourage responsible parenthood and the sanctity of human life.

Finally a personal comment, a statement of faith. As father of two healthy sons and one son whose life was taken early, I have a small understanding of the mysterious goodness of life when contrasted to death. I feel we should choose life with all the strength God gives us. Remember the words of Pearl Buck, whose retarded daughter was the strength of her life: "Beyond life lie only faith and surmise, but not knowledge. Where there is no knowledge except for life, decision for death is not safe for the human race."[27]

# 6. Rebuilding Man

We have explored two problems related to control over germinal and perinatal life. Here technologies prevail with great power over the human life: potential or nascent. The decision-making contexts of heart replacement, organ replacement, cyborg medicine, and the broad area of rebuilding man are all situations where human energy and mechanical energy are joined in lively interaction.

There is a long history of comparing man to, and contrasting him with, the machine. The recent fields of biomathematics, biomechanics, and bioengineering are outgrowths of this quest. If all human functions are able to be understood in mathematical formulae, according to the basic laws of physics, then, it is contended, human functions can be mechanically modeled and finally replaced by an artifact. The organs are pumps; the limbs are levers; the brain, a computer.

How do we evaluate the ethical use of this understanding and technical implementation? In one sense we are dealing with a commendable effort to sustain vitality in a person when replaceable functions fail. The radio control impulse which removes the foot-dragging necessity in a person who has had a cerebral vascular accident is an example. The artificial sphincter muscle that restores a semblance of continence to a spina bifida child is another. But where does the process of rebuilding man into a machine become absurd? When is the desire to make a machinelike man a perverted quest for physical immortality? We know the modern plastics are indestructible. Does that mean that we will fabricate a plastic man in order to achieve immortality? In submitting the activity of rebuilding man to ethical analysis, we will consider the human heart replacement as a clinical microcosm. The heart is the throbbing center of life. When it fails, all else collapses.

On April 3, 1969, Dr. Denton Cooley, medical director of the Texas Heart Institute in the Texas Medical Center, replaced the diseased heart of Haskell Karp with a completely artificial heart.[1] A flurry of criticism followed. Significantly, the public excitement did not reach the level it had in December 1967 when Dr. Christian Barnard performed the first human homo transplant. The reasons for this were several. The first instance of the total excising of a human heart had already occurred numerous times. This was merely another instance. In addition to this, the ethical and moral sensibilities of man are not so offended by artifact substitution as they are by human donation. Pacemakers, synthetic vascular grafts, and artificial valves have long been widely utilized. The artificial heart was merely another prosthetic reduplication of cardiovascular function.

The operation was new and innovative. Perhaps it was premature in light of incomplete animal studies and related research. Very likely it was a trial of procedure that will be commonplace in another ten years. It stood, however, in a long sequence and broad context of cardiac procedure. Far from being radically innovative, the event was a natural step in the evolutionary development of biomedical advance. It stood in the stream of endeavor to replace and reduplicate diseased human organs. It was part of the heroic enterprise of medical intervention in cardiac disease. It reflected the strong commitment of civilized man to salvage and rebuild the man who is functionally debilitated.

Karp died, as did most of the pioneer recipients in the first months of human heart replacement. Perhaps a pessimism has set in. The inrush of anxious candidates for a transplant has subsided. The cardiac units of the great medical centers are not filled with expectant patients waiting to hear the scream of the ambulance siren. This was the situation just months ago. Karp and his physician had no choice. He was a desperately sick man. He dared to risk. He lost. We now know that he contributed in his death to a growing scientific knowledge. A growing conviction is felt today among those expert in the field that the great promise of prosthetic replacement of the human heart deserves the continued commitment of public resource.[2]

Since the burden of illness in the West has shifted from communicable disease to degenerative disease, the problem of a premature heart failure is a major one. Although it is a larger problem in the affluent Occidental lands than elsewhere in the world, it looms universally as a great force harming and killing man. Coronary failure takes nearly three-quarters of a million lives each year in the United States alone. This figure constitutes at least 50% of mortality statistics. Great alleviation of this social blight is promised by emerging skills in medicosurgical treatment of cardiovascular disease and the prospect of successful styles of human heart replacement.

The issues of human heart replacement deserve thoughtful and objective attention. The purpose of this chapter is to place the current and contemplated procedures in a moral perspective and to appropriate the insight of ethical science to these questions. Whereas the themes of creativity and procreativity, understandings of man's task on the earth, were organizing motifs in the last chapter, the issues of *freedom* and *coercion* will provide framework for this evaluation. The dynamic interplay of values in this decision-making context lend themselves to evaluation under these themes.

The chapter will move in two stages. First, the clinical data will be surveyed in the light of the motifs of coercion and freedom. Finally, an attempt will be made to relate our working decision-making model in a way which will minimize coercion and maximize freedom. I prefer to describe this final section as a sketch of an ethical guideline which keeps the decision-making context humane.

My clinical experience is confined to the Texas Medical Center. Here at the Methodist and St. Luke's Hospitals there have been more than thirty implants to date. The center has performed more human heart replacements than any other center in the world. This fact has given rise to many confusing arguments. When Dr. Cooley performs four implants in three days, regional "Texas" style is questioned. Professional and hospital jealousies come into play. The dramatic, stagelike publicity surrounding these events has clouded the profound central issues. This chapter will not concentrate on, nor avoid, these considerations.

We have had one heterograft (sometimes referred to as Xenograft). A ram's heart was used in an extreme emergency situation where no acceptable human donor was available.[3] We have had numerous allografts. We have had the single artificial implant. This clinical experience, coupled with reading in the medical, psychiatric, and pastoral literature on the subject, is the basis of this reflection.

*Clinical Data:*

In order to accord coercion a meaningful reflection from an ethical point of view, it is necessary to scrutinize some of the clinical data using the concepts of coercion and freedom. The donor situations are particularly prone to the coercive violation of freedom. An instance of this kind occurred in Houston in 1969. A young man had committed suicide after a game of Russian roulette. His relatives were approached by staff seeking his heart for a recipient waiting in an adjacent hospital. In shock, the family refused. The newspaper announced that evening that the family had denied consent to use his organ. This instance certainly was more blunder than malice, but it points to the fact of coercion by threat in these situations. Threat can be explicit, expressed, or merely felt. It is very difficult for a surgeon and his team to request an organ from relatives of one who is dying. This situation, charged with fear, guilt, and dread, makes a coercionless request impossible. Often the "What if I don't?" question carries the threat.

Another more vivid instance of the coercive dynamics involved is expressed in the sibling donor situation in renal transplantation.[4] Cases are on record indicating the onset of severe emotional crisis after a person refused to donate a kidney. Our Institute was recently involved in a situation which concerned four brothers who could have saved the fifth brother's life by donating a kidney if they could have overriden the adamant refusal of their four wives.

The mystique and power of the doctor also carries a coercive possibility to decision-making in extremis. The tension-filled dialogue of Dr. Christian Barnard and his first transplant patient, Louis Washkansky, is often repeated: "Dr. Barnard had already told Washkansky what he had in mind, adding, 'You can have two days to think it over.' Washkansky decided in two minutes: 'Go ahead.' "[5] Decisions at this juncture are often made as desperately weary patients submit themselves to the expertise and authority of the physician. The ethical question that rises here concerns the culpability of a physician who makes a choice when a patient is unconscious or rationally unable to weigh options. Dr. Cooley decided to use the first artificial implant after Karp was open on the table, although Karp desired another procedure. When the transplant proved unfeasible, the decision was made on the basis of the submission to authority previously rendered. The coercion of this procedure is ambivalent, of course, and litigation initiated by Mrs. Karp has been settled out of court.[6]

The classic philosophical distinction of variance or contradiction of wills which control the concepts of freedom and coercion is difficult to apply to this medical context. Here a long process of disease and striving for health has brought the will of physician and patient to coincide. In fact, in this day of anesthetics and powerful chemotherapy, it may be necessary to speak of the eradication of the patient's conscious will as it is rendered submissive to the authority in whose hands one had placed his life, namely, the physician. Hope to avert this dilemma may be afforded by new pain drugs which retain clear consciousness in the patient.

Coronary disease and the value-fraught decision-making of that sphere create a difficult type of situation. Man in cardiac failure is man in extremis. Never before has medical treatment afforded such a Lazarus-like experience. The patient literally sinks into the grave through the long process of illness. Father Damian, the French Dominican priest, was totally disabled after a series of heart attacks. After his transplant, he could jog two miles a day. The prospect of a heart transplant literally holds out the hope of being lifted out of the grave.[7] Irvin Kraft, the psychiatrist with the St. Luke's team, notes the euphoric feeling in the new world that the hospital became for these desperately ill people. The world had been passing them by. The incapacitating disease had rendered most of them "basket cases." Now in the hospital setting, they found a new social system and value system which brought status and respect. Some gloried in the publicity. One man had a bulletin board of clippings. Renewed hope surged in this newly formed commune.[8]

A desperation also invaded the environment. One who received a heart would become sick. He was removed from the unit before he died. The other patients were told, quite correctly, that it was pneumonia or something other than the new heart that caused his death. But the terrifying word "rejection" was whispered throughout the unit.[9] The extremis environment is distorted in both directions, rendering rational, noncoerced decision-making difficult, if not impossible. The healing team also finds itself in a crisis situation. The family, physician, nurse, religious counselor, all find this extremis situation demanding in terms of the decisions required of them. A tense and therefore potentially coercive situation existed when the family of Clive Haupt was asked to donate his heart to be implanted into Dr. Blaiberg. Haupt's bride of three months collapsed in shock, and decision had to be rendered by his mother-in-law, a situation involving a complex of coercive elements, you must admit.

Frequently, legal and religious complications add to the fabric of coercion in these settings. Of great interest, but little consequence, were two reported instances where the recipient family asked if the heart of the donor was "saved" or if "Jesus was in his heart."[10] The superstitious aspect of a religious scruple was expressed in at least three cases where the donor was black. Although Dr. Blaiberg himself vigorously avoided it, I have letters which question the "rightness" of putting the "black heart" of Clive Haupt into the "Jewish" body of Philip Blaiberg.

Another way in which the religious factor influenced the context includes the belief on the part of the donor families that "they achieve immortality by donating the heart of a family member."[11] This fact gives rise to demands made by donor families of recipient which will be considered later.

The religious factor is strong throughout the heart replacement experience. An almost primitive perception of the rhythms of mother earth as she throbs a message of fate is evidenced. Deep, traumatic perceptions of providence, judgment, grace, and hope are regularly seen. A turn of events is frequently read as an omen. In summary, a religious intensity pervades the context of cardiac replacement which further complicates in coercive ways the decision-making process.

Legal factors also come to bear on decisions made in this setting. All the parties confronted with choice are aware of ramifications of the law. With donor and recipient there are cost factors which may necessitate litigation. (Who pays for the travel, hospital expense, preparation expense of the donor?) Families are concerned with details of wills and litigation that might ensue in settling an estate. Doctors and nurses have the threat of law hanging over their heads for either negligence or for some positive intervention that may be challenged. Hospital administrators are concerned with court costs in resolving payment in these expensive circumstances.

It should be clear that the clinical setting of human heart replacement is a complex context of decision-making where factors of trauma and urgency greatly complicate a situation when the profound imperatives demand clarity. If we define coercion as any factor which impinges upon one's willful decision, we are clearly dealing with a many-faceted context of coercion. Persons making decisions here are faced with circumstantial environmental coercion, as well as with the various modes of interpersonal coercion.

*Freedom:*

The dynamics of freedom are also present in this clinical experience. In her symposium on freedom, Ruth Nanda Anshen has noted the variety of understandings of freedom in our collected wisdom. All affirm "the autonomy of the rational being developing to ripe maturity and achieving self-fulfillment."[12] I would like to analyze freedom of choice in this crisis setting in this rather basic way. In a tension-fraught clinical setting it is necessary to postulate positive freedoms both to understand what is going on and what should go on—to interpret descriptively as well as normatively. Three understandings of freedom are operative in the heart replacement experience. For the sake of brevity we will label them (a) rational, (b) vital, and (c) altruistic freedom. Although the three understandings intersect and intermingle, it will help our analysis of the decision-making context to distinguish them.

(A) We might define freedom as the capacity of the involved party (donor, recipient, family, physician, etc.) to make a fully rational, informed decision. This freedom to responsible decision is a cardinal tenet of medical practice at its best. This principle undergirds all of the concern of medicoethical literature regarding informed consent. In this situation the patient, in concert with his physician, spouse, spiritual adviser, together with the support of all significant others, analyzes the facts, weighs the alternatives, and renders decision for this or that course of action with full cognizance of possible consequences and the odds. One could say in this situation, "I am free only when I have adequate information, clear mind, and the normal exemption from contradiction in the cause-effect process." Within this view of freedom as clear-minded, informed control, coercion would occur when deception or manipulation took place. If the physician makes a diagnosis or prognosis easy to swallow against the face of truth, he would violate the patient, who had this understanding of freedom.

This type of rational, informed awareness is, of course, impossible with a procedure that is still as much experimental as therapeutic. We have not had enough cases or time lag to project in a meaningful way the possible course of the illness. The initial experience of heart transplantation has been disappointing for all except the recipients who have gained a new lease on life, however brief.

The uncertainties involved impose limitation on freedom. Several people had liquidated their assets, packed up, left home, and moved to a medical center to wait for a transplant only to have to return home when no donor appeared. This "big if" along with the related variable factor of tissue match create uncertainties that make secure planning and decision-making difficult. Freedom in this sense demands a predictability factor which is frequently not present in these cases.

The activity of drug therapy also comes to bear on this understanding of freedom. If therapeutic intervention of any type makes it impossible for this man to participate in deciding his future, freedom, thus understood, has been compromised. Both radical pain and drugs distort clear thought. The delicate consideration of both factors seems necessary to protect this freedom.

One of the potential issues in the area of the artificial heart bears focusing on this point. If a mechanical heart is placed in the body of a man, the energizing force is no longer linked to the regulating mechanisms of his central nervous system but rather to an independent power source. In this sense, both a pacemaker and a cardiac prosthesis work outside of man's control. One of the physiological problems of this device is that of accelerating or quieting the heart rhythms when body function demands this. The ethical concern is related to the large concerns of cyborgs in general.[13] How much human activity should be mechanically reduplicated? When is man controlled by contrived functions he formerly exerted control over? When on the spectrum of the man-machine chimera does man become a machine? The great tragedy of a person with spinal cord injury who becomes quadriplegic is the way rational control over his circumstance is delimited. Perhaps he cannot push a call-button; certainly, he cannot take his life.

(B) Alternatively, freedom might be defined as the extension or enrichment of the act of living. From this perspective, rational control is not so important as saving or lengthening life. Whatever it takes is legitimate. Drug therapy, radical surgery, even loss or diminution of function (i.e., amputation, lobotomy) is justified if some modicum of life is spared. Some feel that it is worth being kept alive even when cerebral responsiveness is gone. "To be free is to be alive. Hopefully to be fully aware, functioning and free from pain, but alive in any case." Anything is justified if any spark of life is maintained. This may fall anywhere on the spectrum that runs from vitality to vegetation. "Man will endure," says Thornton Wilder. But is the quality of durability in a machine a value that should be translocated to man?

Interesting theological comment could be brought to bear on this understanding of freedom. Is mere physical vitality a good of such a high order? Is such desperate clinging to life an act of defiance against God? Two views can be distinguished in the theological literature. *Christianity Today,* a conservative journal, questions this longing for life extension when held up against the promise of resurrection continuity of life.

Man's hope that science may offer temporal immortality, by perpetual replacement of outworn organs, may in fact spring from a perverse rejection of his creaturehood and an aspiration to man-made eternity. The haunting question, to be addressed to those whose present existence is really a living death, is: What do you want a new heart for?[14]

The question is framed differently in Dietrich Bonhoeffer's thought on this question. The tenacious clinging to life is not an expression of faithlessness, says Bonhoeffer, but rather the expression of faith and gratitude in the goodness and importance of man's time on earth. In an advent (1943) letter to a friend he writes:

It is only when one loves life and the earth so much that without them everything would be gone, that one can believe in the resurrection and a new world.[15]

It is interesting that these two theological statements base the ethical imperative of grasping onto life on the resurrection. Both emphases are present in the tradition of Christian theology. They are both expressed at the human emotional level in this clinical experience. Although there could be no documentation on this point, it is my impression that those who believe that this life is "all there is" cling more tenaciously to life and make better postoperative progress in heart replacement situations than do those who have various shades of belief in afterlife. The pastoral evidence, however, is mixed. Some contend that the peace and composure of genuine resurrection confidence promotes healing and recovery more than "frantic attempts" to hold onto what you have.[16]

When freedom is understood in this vitalistic way, coercion occurs when measures of euthanasia or antidysthanasia take place. Coercion is likewise involved when forms of human experimentation serve the purpose of medical knowledge at the expense of the patient's life. When we raise the normative question of whether one is wrong to place his life in such an experimental situation when this knowledge might help future generations, we approach the third understanding of freedom.

(C) The act of altruism is often the principle around which one's freedom understanding is built. One could argue that the personal decision or act that most fully serves one's fellowman is the most creative of freedom. This factor of the "greater love" (John 15:13) is frequently present in the donation act of heart transplantation. This motivation sustains the two strong organ donation programs that have begun.[17]

The altruistic motive is also involved in the recipient act. "If this decision will serve the emerging scientific knowledge and eventually save the lives of others," goes the argument, "it is good and responsible to take the chance even if death ensues." If freedom is thus defined, coercion is present in legal and religious scruples which limit the donation of organs. The Neuremberg experience and literature show this "delayed benefit" value taken to absurd conclusion. Hundreds of experimental victims were sacrificed for the dubious goal of scientific knowledge that would benefit future generations. For this reason the code warns that "the degree of risk to be taken should never exceed that determined by the humanitarian importance of the problem to be solved by the experiment" (Principle Number 6).

One interesting potential problem concerns the question of whether we can forbid someone to donate an organ, even a heart. While Mr. Karp lay critically ill, the hospital received a call saying that a heart would be made available if fifty thousand dollars were deposited in a designated bank. A wealthy Canadian says he will appear at a Toronto hospital with a kidney donor. Perhaps men will soon sell their hearts to feed a hungry family or pay a debt. Perhaps a new organ "black market" will recall the horrors of the nineteenth century. The altruistic aspect in tissue donation should be encouraged and legally facilitated before this unfortunate practice begins.[18]

## The Decision-making Model:

In a pluralistic society the ethical model we have constructed would seem to facilitate the freedoms enumerated and diminish the coercions. In this model personal and social values are balanced. The great danger in our present passion to rebuild man, reflected for example in the decision to cover dialysis under social security, is its neglect of retrospective and prospective insight. I have elsewhere related this concern to Huxley's "higher utilitarianism."[19] Certainly, the wisdom of experience and the weighing of consequences must come to refine our current fascination with the medically exotic problem.

We presently invest large amounts of money in treatment of the rare and isolated cases and neglect the broader social imperatives. What an indictment on disordered human priorities are poor Mississippi blacks or Calcutta outcasts witnessing the news of another heart transplant while their children starve to death before their very eyes.

The opening words of Dr. Henry Beecher before the Senate committee hearing on the "Mondale" proposal summarize the author's feelings in this section: "Transplantation of the heart represents a desperate effort to save a desperate situation. The same is true of the artificial heart. In my judgment, these therapeutic attempts to help a dying man are proper and ethical."[20]

In conclusion, let me merely enumerate some guidelines that would be indicated by our analysis and would serve to humanize the decision-making context of heart replacement.

*Guidelines:*

(A) Media coverage of heart replacement should attempt balanced reporting. Wherever possible, the therapeutic efforts should be allowed the thoughtful scrutiny of the scientific literature before detailed analytic material is released to the public media. The coverage should not allow the extremes of unwarranted optimism or pessimism to control the reporting.[21] There was something misleading in the romanticized portrayal of transplant recipients swimming off the Cape of Good Hope, or playing golf in Phoenix, selling cars in Houston. Not that the lease of life given these men was less than miraculous. The courage of hospital teams as well as patients was an inspiration to people around the world. The problem, as Mrs. Blaiberg later disclosed, was that the romanticism distorted the picture. Beneath the exuberant and energetic life caricatured by the press was a "hell-like" ordeal, full of terror. The distorted media coverage only raised expectations which could never be fulfilled, as well as painting a rose-colored picture not quite true to facts.

The physician's sensibilities are important at this point. Christian Barnard's announcement to the press (CBS News, March 20, 1970) that he plans to do a brain transplant is not helpful, in that it raises inappropriate expectations.

(B) A second guideline that would serve to humanize the context of heart replacement would call for the giving of all possible information so that the "reasoned consent" freedom of man is protected. The physician who "tells it like it is" with thoughtful thoroughness, avoiding the extremes of optimistic or pessimistic exaggeration, is to be commended.

(C) Donation situations should be kept as free from coercion as possible. This is a two-sided concern. There should be more education, wider knowledge of programs like the Living Bank, nationwide adoption of an even stronger tissue donation statute, so that organ donation is facilitated.[22] Counsel should also be given donor families to be less compulsive in the demands they make on recipients.[23]

(D) Protecting the rights of the recipient requires continued refinement of thought and increased loyalty to humane guidelines of human experimentation.

(E) Freedom and coercion are good concepts against which to evaluate a decision-making context. The ideal context is one where all signals are responded to. There are normative signals that proceed from man's historic experience and spiritual insight into what is good. These signals constitute the retrospective source of ethical insight. There are relational signals that move among the parties involved in a given crisis situation. These constitute the introspective insight. There are signals from the future. I call these feedback or prospective signals. Their message concerns what will happen if we choose or fail to choose a certain course of action. All of these signals have personal and socioenvironmental dimensions. Any humane decision will be responsive to all the signals that reverberate through the context. Directives proceed from our history, the future, the network of relatedness. This is the way man perceives the will of God: "I face the One in the actions of the many upon me,"[24] writes H. Richard Niebuhr.

Let us illustrate the use of our decision-making model by examining the question our nation must decide in the area of the artificial heart. The national task force pondering all of the ramifications of this technology has long struggled with this problem. Is the development of an artificial heart a high order national priority? Is it an urgent necessity worthy of a space program or cancer conquestlike effort? Should mechanisms of diagnosis be made mandatory under national insurances, say for young men who might have arteriosclerotic build up, A-type personality and thus run the high risk of myocardial infarction? Should an implant be required of such persons as a condition to remaining insurable?

In all these questions deep insights emerge along the three vectors we have discussed. The nature of man, historically discerned, reveals that he is a creature who defies mechanization yet craves long and full life. These insights will prompt us to utilize the technology of the artificial heart only in those cases where premature heart crisis cuts short a life still having great potential. The introspective insights will search out the psychodynamics and interpersonal interactions which render this procedure wholesome or absurd. The sociopolitical structures which facilitate equitable accessibility to this procedure or the perpetuation of the prevailing unjust distribution patterns also become clear in this analysis. Will blacks and other indigent Americans who populate the publically financed teaching hospitals of our land continue to be not only the exploited experimental population but the group deprived of those benefits that ultimately accrue from their willingness to experiment?

Thus the signals from the future can be recorded. Will the widespread use of this technology inflict other forms of suffering? Will it really serve a human good? Research now on the difference in mortality and morbidity statistics with new intensive care units as opposed to older more simple units reveals very little significant improvement, indicating a value disproportionate to the investment. Will the introduction of the artificial heart merely do away with one form of death and thus necessitate death by more refined, excruciating, lingering sickness?

In all of these considerations the choices are highly ambivalent. No development is an unmixed blessing. A full-orbed consideration of the issues will surely make the final decision more humane though not perfect.

In conclusion, a theologian must emphasize the high nobility of giving life to another person by donating the heart. That the heart is the focus of life is not mere poetic jibberish. The heart has a power and transphysical meaning. The beating of a living heart, like the electric impulses of the central nervous system, is a miraculous power at once mechanical and yet somehow close to the quick of life itself.

Anyone who has spent any time in cardiovascular surgery knows the inordinate strength of this organ when viable. To treat it surgically is to hold life in one's hands. To replace it is to give life itself. To even think about the effort of heart replacement is in itself a biomedical and spiritual exercise.

Rebuilding man, as exemplified in this replacement of the physiological center of his vitality, is an activity where man's creative life energy confronts all the terror of his finitude. Here man is forced to affirm value greater than his personality. Dobzhansky writes:

. . . Man knows that he is mortal, and this brings forcibly the perception of his radical finitude. The finitude becomes more bearable only when he accepts himself as a constituent part of an ongoing operation—mankind—which may move toward eternity.[25]

# 7. Controlling Man

Of all the problems of medical ethics the one that most clearly shows the need for comprehensive moral framework is that of brain and behavior control. A range of procedures is involved, from education to direct electrical and surgical intervention with intermediate measures like psychological conditioning and subliminal persuasion. Parties exercising mind control range from medical doctors to psychological counselors to political leaders. Although clear distinctions must be made between clinical treatment of psychomotor epilepsy and television advertising as techniques of behavior modification, it is desirable to establish the broad ethos where all such activities can be evaluated. We need to note initially how the human brain is brought into the sphere of technical control. Following a brief description of the problems, we will need to search the retrospective, introspective, and prospective paths of ethical insight to derive the norms for presently used and designed methods of control.

There is no doubt that we stand today at the threshold of the "final revolution."[1] Aldous Huxley used this phrase to characterize the day when technology would be applied not only to matter but to man. Today, writers like B. F. Skinner[2] and Michael Crichton[3] and films like *Charlie, Clockwork Orange,* and *The Ruling Class* ask us to weigh the morality of applying technical control to the human brain. Psychobiological and pharmacological means of personal manipulation in concert with electronic media and mass communications as tools of social persuasion create an ambiguous future of promise and threat. The personal significance of this development still lies largely in the future. The techniques of therapeutic mind manipulation are still largely limited to the laboratories of men like Professors Delgado and Heath; but the whole range of procedure that Albert Rosenfeld vividly chronicles as electrochemical control of the brain and behavior[4] is now beginning to break in upon us as a powerful issue.

The sociopolitical organs of coercion which control thought and behavior are better known and already operative, education, family, and organized religion having perhaps more positive than malignant effect. Then there are ominous examples: the Stalin era, the recent Czech experience, the latent though perhaps overstated threat of media control in our own country. These, along with the powerful reflective work of Arthur Koestler,[5] certainly make vivid both the potentiality and the actuality of mass mind control.

To survey our problem responsibly we must first note the way in which the human central nervous system comes to be enfolded by what Delgado calls "the experimental reach." Just as in molecular biology where the vitalism assumption of Pasteur assumed that no vital process could occur outside the sacristy of a living cell, so in our cultural history the mind was considered something special, not vulnerable to empirical analysis. The mind was sacrosanct. This conception is shaped by the Greek body/mind dualism that infiltrates our religious history and the mind/matter distinction that has controlled our philosophic tradition since Descartes.

Then one night in the eighteenth century this situation began to change. Mama Galvani was preparing frog legs for her husband Luigi. The couple noted the way the legs twitched and jumped when hooked on a copper wire. From the time of Galen in second-century A.D. Greece, men believed that there was a spirit, an *anima,* that activated neurologic impulse. Galvani's frog legs began a long process of discovery in which men came to see nervous system function in terms of electrical and chemical process.

Today the disciplines of neurophysiology, psychopharmacology, and cybernetics reflect the advance of this developing understanding of the dynamics of mentation. It is this history which frames the theme of this chapter: technical manipulation of the brain.

The problem is at least tripartite:[6] we must first consider direct manipulation of the brain through surgical, chemical, and electrical means. There is the direct intervention into an individual's central nervous system, which can occur through psychosurgery, chemical modification of behavior, and implanting electrodes or otherwise initiating or simulating the electrical activities of the brain. This initial capacity enables us to heighten or diminish cerebral activity through a surgical, chemical, or electrical intervention into the brain's functioning. We are now able, or soon will be able, to relieve pain, stimulate pleasure, intensify or eradicate memory, provoke sexual activity, control anger, induce euphoria.

Psychosurgery is a theme provoking wide controversy today. It involves excising certain portions of the brain to limit the effect of harmful lesions. Prefrontal lobotomy to relieve the effects of severe depressive psychosis is an example of the technique. Dr. Luria, Russia's renowned brain physiologist, believes that many behavior aberrations are caused by brain lesions. Following localization of the lesion through interviewing, psychosurgery is recommended to correct, for example, a learning disorder. Some suggest legally required psychosurgery for pathological criminals. The liberating and potentially threatening dimensions of this capacity are immediately evident.

Chemical manipulation of the brain involves drug-induced alterations of behavior: heightened or diminished awareness via the wide range of stimulants, depressants, and psychotropic agents. The techniques that concern us here introduce the tantalizing prospects of chemical transference of knowledge and experience.

The social ramifications of chemical manipulation are perhaps more ominous than those involving electrical means. Chemical warfare and recent threats from militant circles to detonate charges or drip LSD into a city's water supply illustrate this ominous prospect. To effect a change in human functioning by altering the chemistry of what man ingests or breathes is a frightening capacity.

Secondly, there is the activity of reduplicating or extending central nervous system activity with the machine, principally with the computer. This cybernetic capacity enables us to extend the central nervous system into the world. The machine enlarges the power of the human brain, extending its activity through anticipation planning, decision-making, and feedback analysis. In this activity man harnesses more of the cosmic energies to the nexus of his brain. He thus transforms reality into what authors have variously called "the global electronic village"[7] or "noosphere."[8]

The very common forms of mind manipulation are vivid and need no enumeration. Often we ignore them and fail to see the extent of their control. Needs are created according to vested interests. Through advertising, political ideology is introduced and enforced. Patterns of perceiving and thinking are altered in the feedback cycles initiated as human extensions create environments.

To consider these matters in a religioethical context necessitates a look at the Judeo-Christian anthropology, particularly the facets of that anthropological tradition which bears on concerns of the mind.

In Hebrew thought man's mind is the profound level of perception which springs from his unified biospiritual being.

Hebrew man feels, knows, and perceives in one unitive act (*Lev; Col,* i.e., Psalm 26:2, and *krev,* Psalm 64:6). The Hebrew verb for knowledge is also used for human intercourse. In other words, the essence of the Hebrew understanding of mind is relatedness: relatedness to God, to man, to Torah. The mind, in other words, is the mystical, rational, and emotional contact man has with objective reality and *Thou.*

In the Greek world notions of reason, mind, *logos,* are refined and sharpened. Man's mind can be the instrument of his glory or his hubris, expressing either his ascent or his fall, depending on one's answer to the Tertullian question, "What has Athens to do with Jerusalem?"

In Greek wisdom man's reason is his link with the rational nature of things. It may be a divine spark of spirit, *pneuma*, as in Stoicism, or the structural soul as in Aristotle, *psuche nous.* Underlying this differentiation is the belief that mind is the capacity guiding man's perception of reality. Perpetuating this tradition, Rene Dubos sees the mind as the reflection of environmental stimuli. Man is *logikos*, a rational being linked to universal reason. Mind serves to link man to eternal reality (Plato)[9] or structurally to order his being, teleologically drawing personality toward fulfillment and destiny (Aristotle).

From these roots Jewish and Greek emerges the Christian understanding of mind, soul, and conscience. In Christian tradition the consciousness of man in cognitive, emotive, and ethical aspect is only deepened and complicated rather than simplified.

Before valuative statements can be made concerning mind manipulation, we must grapple with this problem. What entity or function called "mind" is or should be unmanipulatable, and why? What situations justify the use of brain control? The classic philosophic reflection on the mind-body interface seems to have lost its intrigue.[10] We can talk about the mind structurally or functionally. Each perspective offers different ethical directives. If we focus structurally, biological intervention might be most objectionable. If we conceive of the mind functionally, either in Freudian personality terms of ego, superego, etc., or philosophically, in terms of freedom, responsibility, etc., a different constellation of values becomes normative.

The subject of "mind" generally has been reviewed from at least three perspectives. Neurophysiologists and psychopharmacologists stress the brain as system, activated by electrochemical and psychic process. Philosophers stress mental qualities: freedom, choice, responsibility. This tradition runs deep in philosophy through Kant's delineation of pure and practical reason, back to Plato and Aristotle. Although each of these emphases, the structural and functional, emerges in Christian history, the unique contribution of theological thought is to see the ethical reality of mind.

In Christian anthropology man's uniqueness resides not in his brain, majestic and marvelous as it is, nor in his reason. Theology finds the grandeur and uniqueness of man's mind in his reason, located in his responsibility. Relatedness, personal responsiveness to another, *verantwortung,* answerability, communicativeness between man and God, man and man—these factors constitute the mental genius of man. Man is more than an animal, even a rational animal. He is a moral being, a responsive, responsible, creature. Emil Brunner, for example, stresses that reason is not an entity but a relation.[11] Ethically speaking, man is a man only when he can personally relate and decide. Humanness is active in the presence of interpersonal, intrapsychic, and transcendent relatedness and in the exertion of moral discernment.

The components of the Judeo-Christian tradition highlight different aspects of mind. Roman Catholic thought accents the organic nature of mind. Jewish theology is focused on the rational aspects of mind. In Protestant thought the relational stress is made. The unified stream running through the rich tradition, however, is the view that man is a personal being, unique in his capacity to relate as "thou" rather than "it," and his moral capacity to understand and to stand under the Word of God.[12]

Before passing from this section on Judeo-Christian anthropology, we must make reference to the Marxist view of man. There are two reasons for this. First, Marxism is the major secular *weltanschauung* and view of man that Judeo-Christian tradition has spawned. Secondly, the secular humanism of Marxism may well prove to be an appreciated "soul brother" if the world continues to propel itself toward more nihilistic, antihuman ideologies. Marxism emerges in Western philosophy via Hegel. It combats all forms of alienation of man. In the words of Czech scientist Jan Kamaryt, "it [Marxism] is directed against all attempts of reducing man to a manipulable being. This has led . . . to Marx's concept of the free, total and productive man."[13]

Free and deliberate choice is a fundamental quality of man's inner being which is open, always in the process of becoming. These elements of free being and overcoming alienation are cardinal Marxist tenets. We know how frequently they are suspended or abrogated in the socialist state. We can also question whether real mental and soul freedom are possible in a social order which clings to either a-theism or anti-theism as "politically enforced values." Despite these objections and the unfortunate vulnerability of Marxist nations to freedom negation through cybernetic control and planning, we would be wise to move from anathema to dialogue.[14] We should accept and foster the mind humanism of that tradition, as together we face the terror and promise of mind manipulation.

These anthropological insights can be related to the present and potential problems of mind manipulation. It seems important initially to set the ethical context. In our opening section on moral analysis we argued for an ethical decision-making model where the responsible self is sensitive to all the signals that reverberate through the context. This is the rational-relational setting of the Judeo-Christian ethics. One is here responsive to retrospective, introspective, and prospective signals. This ethic is responsive not only to insights from tradition, but also to the present network of relation and mutual effect, and to the future.[15]

Let us take an illustration. We are confronted with a decision to require a surgical or electrical intervention into the mind processes of a person who has fits of violent aggressive behavior. Let us assume that we have the surgical or electrical capacity to modulate this violent behavior into cowlike passive sweetness. The ethical context might be bombarded with signals from behind, ahead, and the sides. Tradition might remind us of the violent capacity engraved in the being of all men in the mark of Cain. It might remind us that "being my brother's keeper" is a matter of free will. In this case we might disallow or justify brain manipulation because he is either *free* or *not free* biologically to be his "brother's keeper." Another normative signal from memory might be the classic restraints on human experimentation. Horizontally or laterally the context might receive signals regarding the social desirability of intervention. Family concerns, public safety, or the common law insight of right of protection from oneself might find meaning in this case.

The signals from the future might include the genetic load prospect if some deleterious trait is not isolated. It might consider the feedback effect of allowing or disallowing this form of mind alteration to occur. All of these factors, retrospective, introspective or circumspective, and prespective, seem to impinge upon any given decision, constituting its ethical context.

Here, I believe, we are approaching what has classically been called the discernment of "the will of God." This certainly is the impetus and directive that is ultimate in any ethic. A strong synthesis of traditionalism, situationalism, and futurism appears to be the only responsible way to act with reference to these great crisis questions. The alternatives are a collapse into fatalism or legalism, faults to which men are perenially prone. These are not ethical options open to responsible men today.

H. Richard Niebuhr in his study of *The Responsible Self* succinctly summarizes the kind of ethic I am opting for. He does it by contrasting responsive ethics to the idealist and legalist options. Monotheistic idealism says, "Remember God's plan for your life." Monistic deontology commands, "Obey God's law in all your obedience to finite rules." Responsibility affirms, "God is acting in all actions upon you. So respond to all actions upon you as you respond to his action."[16]

Accepting this model of a responsiveness ethic in a context open to past, present, and future seems to propose several moral directives regarding this question of mind manipulation. I merely state these in conclusion:

(A) The Gerard thesis that "there can be no twisted thought without a twisted molecule"[17] needs to be understood together with a biblical insight. It comes from Jeremiah: "The heart is deceitful above all things, and desperately corrupt; who can understand it? 'I the Lord search the mind and try the heart' " (17:9–10, RSV). Our mind scientists and therapists should be encouraged in their efforts to heal pathologies that are organic in origin, giving rise to violent behavior. We should not allow ourselves the simplistic view of man, however, which reduces all human evil or good to disturbed electrochemical process. This would deny the richness of human freedom and will, miss the power involved in man's "intentionality,"[18] and distort the spectrum of human activity under God that makes him a man: hate, despair, repentance, love, aspiration. To see these activities as molecular not only in action but in origin would lead to a disastrous anthropology and consequently justify a frightful range of mind manipulation technique. The Gerard statement is fully acceptable unless we interpret it to mean that the twisted molecule is the sole and sufficient cause of the twisted thought. We must allow what Dr. Delgado calls the extracerebral elements of mind. Judeo-Christian ethics would argue that man is a moral being. Although his good and evil intentionality may have organic expression, it is rooted in the way that personal being relates to "the ground of being" and fellow humanity.

The central value of our ethical wisdom at this point is to preserve the moral freedom of man. When physical or chemical impediments exist, thwarting this freedom, the techniques of brain control are certainly justified to return the person to normalcy. The only danger to be avoided is a greater compromise of freedom in the trade-off. But when we hear proposals such as those at a recent meeting of the American Psychological Association which call for ethics pills to transform into benevolence the malice of politicians, we must affirm that we dare not go beyond freedom and dignity.

(B) Dr. Delgado's postulate that "we can intelligently manipulate the cerebral determinants of behavior"[19] prompts an observation and a suggested guideline. I question the assumed *intelligence* of man. Reinhold Niebuhr commented on the way that sinfulness is the most empirically verifiable human fact. Koestler speaks of the strain of insanity that runs through our species. At recent Senate hearings on this subject Senator Walter F. Mondale of Minnesota posed the question, "Are we wise enough to be so smart?"[20] With reference to genetic manipulation Marshall Nirenberg said, "When man becomes capable of instructing his own cells, he must refrain from doing so until he has sufficient wisdom to use this knowledge for the benefit of mankind."[21]

I tend to agree with these notions. Dr. Delgado claims that our scientific progress has a momentum that cannot be halted or reversed. He expressed the well-founded fear of Robert Oppenheimer that what is technically sweet becomes irresistible. Delgado phrases his pessimism this way:

It would be irrelevant to discuss whether physical control of the mind should be accepted or rejected since history proves that when technology has been available, it has been used and developed regardless of possible dangers or moral issues.[22]

Although history certainly bears out the argument, we cannot allow ourselves to slip into fatalism. Although Delgado's statement has been true in the past, it need not be true for us. We can say no to alluring avenues of research. Our universities can refuse government grants. We can exert political influence to prevent destructive use of our technology. With Norbert Wiener we can refuse to give research insight to irresponsible militarists.[23] We can develop scientific conscience in the life sciences as physicists attempt to do in the *Bulletin of Atomic Scientists*. Fortunately, a profound moral consciousness is emerging in the scientific community. This is evidenced by the humanistic direction of distinguished scientists around the world. The dynamic understanding of personality, forged in the crucible of Jewish and Greek anthropology, cherished in the Judeo-Christian ethic, would call us to creative aspiration, not acquiescence. The traditional elements of historical openness, meaningful progress, and hope prompt us to use our science and technology for human fulfillment rather than for destruction.

Our future is open. It throbs with human responsibility because it is God's future. Karl Rahner states it succinctly:

In the obviously growing openness to the future and its planning . . . the dialectic of increased planning and unplanned contingency . . . God's absolute future perhaps shows itself in silent presence.[24]

We stand at the threshold of "the final revolution." Psychocivilization is beginning to break in upon us. The promise is evident. Pain, suffering, the great environmental problems, hunger, war, all intensify in world civilization as challenges that cannot be answered without "intelligent technology." Man cannot survive on earth without his science and technology: that is clear. The question is, Can he survive with his technology?

# 8. Immortalizing Man

Our inquiry now moves to the point in a man's life where his vitality begins to fail. To sustain debilitated and failing human life, we draw on many types of technologies and mechanisms. Achieving an ethical quality of life in an age of advanced biotechnology requires an apparent paradoxical commitment. On the one hand, the good requires that we affirm the life impulse in men and energetically strive to protect life against the intrusion of disease and death. On the other hand, we must receive death graciously if man is to have a future. This acceptance of death impulse is imperative if we are to have good life today and tomorrow. These introspective and prespective insights provide the surest guidelines for our decision-making. The dimension of human reality shaped by organ replacement and biological death affords a context in which to work out man's paradoxical commitment.

Paddy Chayefsky's play *Gideon* is a struggle of a simple man with God but also a struggle of life against death. The Lord, appropriately played by Fredric March, struggles with Gideon. By cunning device three hundred cowardly Israelites with lanterns and rams horns smite the ten thousand armed Midianites. Gideon is the instrument of the Lord. But the Lord demands the death of the Israelite elders who have prostituted life to the way of Moab. Gideon refuses to kill the elders. "I pity them, my Lord," he cries.

"Oh Gideon," says the angel, "you make so much of death. You must not
be so temporal. It is all right for the bulk of men to fear death, for in death
they fear me. But, in truth, there isn't anything to it at all. Nothing happens,
nothing changes; the essence of things goes on. You see, you measure things
in time, but there is no time in truth. You live now ten million years ago and
are at this moment ten million years hence, or more; for there are no years.
The slaying of seventy-seven elders happens but it does not happen, for they
live even so and have and before, and all is now, which was and is forever.
Oh, dear, I see this is heavy going for you."[1]

Two energies activate human life. We oversimplistically call one
creative and one destructive. Understood *sub specie aeternitatis* both
must be creative. There is a life energy that pulses through human
reality. It is found at all levels of life. It struggles to move, it gasps
for breath, it yearns for communion, it defies the intrusions of disease
and death. This impulse is primordially expressed in the locomotive
energy of the amoeba or the phototropic energy of plankton. The
energy is expressed in the fluttering of a decapitated chicken or the
throbbing of an aborted human fetus. Life, especially life imbued with
awareness, struggles for life against death. The life energy is intense
in man. Man yearns to live.

The other energy is the death impulse. Darwin and Freud both
noted the death mechanisms in nature. Whether it be the species'
instinct for survival or the organism's inherent drive toward death, all
life is informed with the principle of destruction. Neo-Freudian disease theorists like David Bakan, for example, show the way that death
is the central teleology of life.[2] Brain neurons die, blood cells destruct,
organs have a life time. The mechanisms of aging have the essential
evolutionary purpose of insuring the future. Even disease, thus understood, functions as a creative condition of life. In this chapter I will
use these two poles of human energy, the life impulse and the death
impulse, as foci by which to interpret the phenomena of organ replacement and biological death. I propose also to use this polarity to focus
the ethical analysis.

*Life Impulse:*

The life energy, or to use Erich Fromm's nondichotomized term, biophilia, is the force that has propelled us to our present position in the life sciences and medical practice. It is impossible to understand the enormous resource that has been poured into biomedicine in the last twenty-five years apart from life energy sustaining the rational quest to know and the emotive quest to defeat death. Clinical transplantation proceeds from this impulse. Tremendous energy is now at work, motivating clinical medicine to repair and sustain failing life. When we concern ourselves with biomedical capacities to immortalize man, we deal with procedures such as organ replacement and prolongation of life. Our biomedical energies are now concerted in effort to defeat the forces that disease debilitate and destroy man. The ultimate consequence of these negative life-salvaging values is the positive value of immortalizing man. Allotransplantation is a widely practiced procedure. Prosthetic replacement and artificial organs offer new promise. Autotransplantation or the innovative procedure of bench surgery provides yet another possibility. These techniques channel rich human and material resources to the goal of rebuilding man.

*Allotransplantation:*

Unless radical breakthroughs occur in our control of tissue histocompatibility, homografts rather than heterografts offer the only hope in human organ replacement.[3] We can expect a limited number of kidney, liver, and heart transplants in the future. These will be limited to the large medical centers and to the rather small number of pathologically exotic people who have physical and financial access to these centers. It remains doubtful that hundreds of thousands of such operations could be performed each year.

*Artificial Organs:*

The artificial organs hold more promise. Although immediate chances of modeling the biochemical complexity of the liver is remote, renal and cardiac prosthesis are well within our reach. Bulky dialysis support to diminished paired organ function should one day yield a sophisticated portable, if not implantable, kidney machine. Several models of artificial heart are now being tested. The mechanical problems are not so formidable as the problem of blood destruction.

*Autotransplantation:*

Bench surgery is a technique now at the final stages of animal testing. It involves the removal of a diseased organ, keeping it viable on an organ preservation bench, cleaning, repairing, or reconstructing it, then replacing it in the body. Autotransplantation of the spleen exemplifies this. The procedure might facilitate excising a kidney stone or lung tumor. Dr. Russell Scott, Urology Chief at Baylor College of Medicine and Methodist Hospital in Houston, is very optimistic. "Bench surgery could be a real breakthrough," he says. "Theoretically, the heart, lung or any organ with a simple blood supply can be disconnected, removed, repaired and reimplanted."[4]

These are the immediate technologies of organ repair and replacement at our disposal. The possibility of laboratory induced tissue growths, genetically fashioned clone counter-parts of individuals, the brain-computer chimera—all afford intriguing but only speculative consideration for the activity of rebuilding man. How can we reflect ethically, philosophically, and theologically on this enterprise?

It is the life energy that harnesses the rational and emotive power to develop, deliver, and receive organ replacement. Man resists death, particularly premature death. Just ponder what an upsurge of humanistic power is newly released in human history. Any cursory sense of history makes this astonishingly clear. Classic culture is inhuman by contrast. Even a nineteenth-century philanthropist could not fathom the tremendous concern for human welfare that characterizes our recent history. To care effectively for fellow humanity is such a new possibility. And man does care. All his energies are activated when he is in the presence of suffering. Although in weakness and fall from his truth he isolates pain and insulates himself from human misery, at his best he sees and feels and responds. This humanism is profoundly present in medicine. Even the most crassly materialistic surgeon is fundamentally motivated by compassion. How else can you explain the discipline and superhuman stamina of the transplant team? What but life energy can explain the dynamics of donor party to the transaction? And the exuberant, often naïve hope of the recipient party? We build the hospitals. We pour in enormous amounts of public and private money. All these disparate yet coordinated energies are expressions of the life urge. To give life and to save life are among the most basic impulses in man. The life urge is at once his highest instinctual response and his noblest supernatural grace.

It is around the principle of life energy that introspective values emerge to insure the quality of life in the area of organ replacement. We call the heroic enterprise of organ replacement good because of the life energy.

Choosing life demands responsibility. Beyond abstract analysis of issues, transplantation is a dynamic transaction involving human persons. A sister and brother from Austin, Texas, will soon die from chronic nephritis unless society rescues them. Their financially exhausted family can no longer sustain the $800 monthly bill for dialysis. Society should support this family out of response to the life instinct. This is not a matter of compassion. It is a matter of duty. National legislation will now insure dialysis and in some cases transplantation under medicaid. This is a choosing of life in the midst of death. In this case of genetically transmitted disease, response to life would also prescribe consultation related to sterilization.

Massive clinical evidence could be marshalled in support of organ replacement as a qualitative good. The kidney transplant experience is very encouraging, although the recent dialysis record is not so good. Liver transplantation has enriched the lives of several children. Heart replacement is in a temporary impasse although recent breakthroughs in immuno-suppressive therapy and surgical technique are most promising. The uniform anatomical gift act is enhancing the facility to give life through tissue donation, so long thwarted by unclear law.

The challenge to our civilization will be that of delivering these gifts of life to the far corners of the earth and to the least of these our brothers. Life energy should prompt us to move in depth and breadth of application with generous resource.

Various death perceptions in our culture affect not only transplants but the whole new field of cryobiology. One might question whether physical vitality alone is a good of such a high order. Is such a desperate clinging to life perhaps an act of defiance against God?

I have argued in the rebuilding man chapter that a clinging to life may be an affirmation of faith and a statement that life is good. A theological understanding of the life impulse would affirm man's "raging thirst for life" as noble. Dylan Thomas has cried with humanistic words close to a Christian affirmation saying that old age should rage against the dying of the light.[5]

*Death Impulse:*

The other pole around which we interpret the data and seek ethical analysis is the death energy. In bold spaced type of Freud's original German edition of *Beyond the Pleasure Principle* he wrote: "Tod Ist Das Ziel Alles Lebens" (the goal of all life is death). All life moves reluctantly but relentlessly towards death. The salmon with death dealing energy drive upstream to spawn, then die. In man every red blood cell must die every 120 days if he is to live. Death runs through the midst of life. Man must receive death graciously if he is to have a future.

Death is a profound embarrassment in a culture so activated by life energy. Aversion to death runs deep in American culture. Someone has said that death is obscenity. Discussion of death is as verboten today as sex was thirty years ago. But biological death is the other locus of our theme. In the context of clinical organ replacement life energy is diametrically opposed to death energy.

The most important conceptual work on biological death has been the recent literature on irreversible coma. If brain death can be accepted clinically and decerebrate life be culturally accepted as non-life, we will have made great strides forward. The Harvard Ad-Hoc Committee, chaired by Henry Beecher, has done the pioneering analysis. The criteria are simple:

A patient in this state appears to be in deep coma. The condition can be satisfactorily diagnosed by points 1, 2, and 3 to follow. The electroencephalogram (point 4) provides confirmatory data, and when available it should be utilized. In situations where for one reason or another electroencephalographic monitoring is not available, the absence of cerebral function has to be determined by purely clinical signs, to be described, or by absence of circulation as judged by standstill of blood in the retinal vessels, or by absence of cardiac activity.

1. *Unreceptivity* and *Unresponsitivity*—There is a total unawareness to externally applied stimuli and inner need and complete unresponsiveness—our definition of irreversible coma. Even the most intensely painful stimuli evoke no vocal or other respónse, not even a groan, withdrawal of a limb, or quickening of respiration.

2. *No Movements or Breathing*—Observations covering a period of at least one hour by physicians is adequate to satisfy the criteria of no spontaneous muscular movements or spontaneous respiration or response to stimuli such as pain, touch, sound, or light. After the patient is on a mechanical respirator, the total absence of spontaneous breathing may be established by turning off the respirator for three minutes and observing whether there is any effort on the part of the subject to breathe spontaneously. (The respirator may be turned off for this time provided that at the start of the trial period the patient's carbon dioxide tension is within the normal range, and provided also that the patient had been breathing room air for at least 10 minutes prior to the trial.)

3. *No reflexes*—Irreversible coma with abolition of central nervous system

activity is evidenced in part by the absence of elicitable reflexes. The pupil will be fixed and dilated and will not respond to a direct source of bright light. Since the establishment of a fixed, dilated pupil is clear-cut in clinical practice, there should be no uncertainty as to its presence. Ocular movement (to head turning and to irrigation of the ears with ice water) and blinking are absent. There is no evidence of postural activity (decerebrate or other). Swallowing, yawning, vocalization are in abeyance. Corneal and pharyngeal reflexes are absent.

As a rule, the stretch of tendon reflexes cannot be elicited; i.e., tapping the tendons of the biceps, triceps, and pronator muscles, quadriceps and gastrocnemius muscles with the reflex hammer elicits no contraction of the respective muscles. Plantar or noxious stimulation gives no response.

4. *Flat Electroencephalogram*—Of great confirmatory value is the flat or isoelectric EEG. We must assume that the electrodes have been properly applied, that the apparatus is functioning normally, and that the personnel in charge is competent. We consider it prudent to have one channel of the apparatus used for an electrocardiogram. This channel will monitor the EEG so that, if it appears in the electroencephalographic leads because of high resistance, it can be readily identified. It also establishes the presence of the active heart in the absence of the EEG. We recommend that another channel be used for a noncephalic lead. This will pick up space-borne or vibration-borne artifacts and identify them. The simplest form of such a monitoring noncephalic electrode has two leads over the dorsum of the hand, preferably the right hand, so the EEG will be minimal or absent. Since one of the requirements of this state is that there be no muscle activity, these two dorsal hand electrodes will not be bothered by muscle artifact. The apparatus should be run at standard gains $10\mu v/mm$, $50\mu v/5mm$. Also it should be isoelectric at double this standard gain which is $5\mu v/mm$ or $25\mu v/5mm$. At least ten full minutes of recording are desirable, but twice that would be better.

It is also suggested that the gains at some point be opened to their full amplitude for a brief period (5 to 100 seconds) to see what is going on. Usually in an intensive care unit artifacts will dominate the picture, but these are readily identifiable. There shall be no electroencephalographic response to noise or to pinch.

All of the above tests shall be repeated at least 24 hours later with no change.

The validity of such data as indications of irreversible cerebral damage depends on the exclusion of two conditions: hypothermia (temperature below 90 F [32.2 C]) or central nervous system depressants, such as barbiturates.[6]

I quote this passage from *JAMA* at length because this clinical guideline is the best we can come up with at present. It may have flaws. One of our cardiovascular surgeons in Houston is loyally served by a secretary who had flat EEG for four days. Extreme caution should temper the most certain guidelines. If we are to maintain quality personal and social life, however, death must be received and accepted. This is offensive to our progressive life-oriented culture. We need now to consider the *extensio ad absurdum* of the immortalizing drive: anabiosis.

Roger Ornsten, a five year old Norwegian boy fell into an icy river in 1962 and drowned. He was under water for 22 minutes and was dead for 2 and ½ hours. After drowning his body temperature fell probably below 75°F, a hypothermia which doctors say prevented swift deterioration of his brain. Although apparently DOA at the hospital, Dr. Tone Kvittingen, who reports the incident in the BRITISH MEDICAL JOURNAL, applied artificial respiration with a tube down the windpipe and rhythmic pressure on the chest to force blood circulation. Although nearly two hours had elapsed without a heartbeat, resuscitation continued, including exchange blood transfusions; natural heartbeat suddenly resumed, and although Roger remained unconscious for six weeks, he now is completely recovered with only slight impairment of muscular coordination and peripheral vision.[7] This dramatic recovery has often been repeated with new cardiopulmonary recuscitation techniques.

This case focuses several important issues that are now surfacing in our culture. The issues are cryobiology, cryogenics, and human hibernation. They represent the *reductio ad absurdum* of the mechanization and rationalization of human life. The larger speculative issue raised is the quest for immortality. In recent years a vast literature, factual, semi-fictional, and fictional, has emerged forcing the question as to whether, at long last, the iceman cometh. Previously the theme has been limited to poetry, science fiction, and Rod Serling. Now the theme of cryogenics and anabiosis appears in the predictive and scientific literature. Robert Ettinger's THE PROSPECT OF IMMORTALITY appeared in 1964. A new book by Lucy Kavaler is entitled FREEZING POINT: COLD AS A MATTER OF LIFE AND DEATH. In the interim numerous studies including Herman Kahn's THE YEAR 2000 and Gordon Taylor's THE BIOLOGICAL TIME BOMB have announced the impending possibility of human hibernation in order to cure disease and increase longevity.

Organization and corporations have answered the call. The Life Extension Society in Washington and the Cryonics Society of New York will answer your questions. Juno Inc. in Springfield, Illinois, is testing prototype "time capsules." Continuelife in Latrobe, Pennsylvania, and Cryolife Corporation in Kansas City are preparing the full package. Union Carbide Corporation is testing both cells and chemicals. According to Ettinger's last appearance on the Merv Griffith Show, several bodies are now suspended in liquid nitrogen capsules, with hundreds more signed up.

The issues raised, though speculative and futuristic, are components of our bio-medical commitments precipitating profound ethical questions even if only in anticipation. Consideration of them is important not for immediate guidelines for decision making or policy formation—but for the sake of getting a reading on attitudes for the sake of decisions that the future will demand. Although the problem is not now pressing in the public arena, it calls for perceptive, retrospective, and prospective ethical insight.

### Ethical Issues

Several issues are raised at this point. (A) First there are the general issues of cryogenics and anabiosis. In a culture that is increasingly secular and sensate, to use Sorokin's phrase, the quest for long, full life will be strong. A recent TV series chronicles the desperation of men trying to achieve a reprieve from death as they chase a man with magic blood; *The Immortal.* Herman Kahn in his forcast of THE YEAR 2000 sees this emergent ethos expressed through numerous impending life extension and hibernation procedures.

In Table 23 on "One Hundred Mechanical Innovations Very Likely (90% +) in the Last Third of the Twentieth Century," he lists:

#14   Extensive use of cyborg techniques (Mechanical aids or substitutes for human organs, senses, links or other components).

#19   Human hibernation for short periods (hours or days) for medical purposes.

#35   Human hibernation for relatively extensive periods (months to years) and . . .

#61   widespread use of cryogenics.

In his table 19 (less likely but important possibilities (50/50%), he lists:

#  8   suspended animation for years or centuries.

#13   major rejuvenation and/or significant extension of vigor and life span, say 100–150 years.

Then in Table 20 (ten far-out possibilities), he lists:

#  1   life expectancy extended to substantially more than 150 years (immortality?).

#  9   life time immunization against practically all diseases.[14]

Cryosurgery is now widespread; cryobiology is increasing in use. Sperm, for example, has been frozen for years, remaining viable to impregnate an egg. Although we may hope such esoteric research will go slowly as we move our medical priorities from the vertical to the horizontal in the first part of this decade, this work is inevitably going to surge ahead.

The issue of hibernation and evolution deserves note. It is a strange twist of history that cryogenic capacity has emerged at the very moment of population crisis. We can begin to learn to extend life only now when the imperative is to limit population. The latter imperative requires both decreasing birth rate and maintaining steady death rate unless we choose to have Haldane's society dominated by the elderly, feeble, and maimed.

Extensive cryogenics could indeed rupture the evolutionary process. The Russian cyberneticist Victor Pekelis expresses this radical paradox: "The maximum metabolic stability—immortality—would mean an end of all evolution."[15] In other words, man must die in order that he live.

A third issue raised in the cryogenic specter concerns quantity versus quality of life. Abnormal longevity can be a horrifying prospect if you stop to think about it. And what of the social dimension? How absurd that *some few* should crave and receive a postponed deadline while for others the basic quality of life goes unfulfilled. Dr. Martin Luther King was prophetic in his last sermon in Memphis when he pondered long life, yet chose God's will.

*Reflections:*

Finally, a reflection or two: I'm wondering how a faithful person in a theological sense or a humanistic person in a secular sense can make imput into our society and the global culture as we make decisions and form policy on these issues. Two things come to mind: they correspond to the retrospective and prespective sectors of ethical insight, the prophetic and priestly elements in life: the naming and breaking of the idols, and the vision of truth. The prophetic task would prompt us to call into question the assumption that we are dealing with some "progressive inevitability" which cannot be stopped. Robert Ettinger expresses this defensive longing: "The theologians in good time will decide on all such questions. Or rather, [a second thought] several schools of theologians [divide and conquer] will each evolve a whole series of accommodations to the developing insights of science and the developing pressures of society, in the usual way."[16] Oppenheimer felt the tragedy of the scientific assumption that what is "technically sweet becomes irresistible." Often we operate on the principle, what we can do—we must do. Perhaps the task of faithful men and human men today is to remind us of our mortality. The quest is noble—not for immortality but for wholeness; not for extraterrestrial escape but for terrestrial responsibility. Man is born to die. The power of technology, as Amosoff suggests, merely throws us back to the meaning of the personal. Theologically discerned, man's mortality, his conditionedness, is the clue to his destiny.

But beyond the prophetic task—the saying *No!* to some plastic world of artificial life—is the priestly, proleptic, constructive task— the saying *Yes!* to that which affirms life and value. This mood asserts that human life has meaning and destiny. This significance is anchored in the cosmic process of renewal that we dare call redemption. This constructive task is going to demand two things of responsible men in the years ahead: Time immemorial has called us to affirm life in the midst of death. Now the future calls us to affirm life in the midst of life.

Quality of life is rooted in its relatedness. I have argued elsewhere for a definition of human relatedness that recognizes intrapsychic and transcendent awareness in addition to stimulus-response and interpersonal relatedness.[17] When these fundamental and profound levels of relatedness are gone, it is categorically immoral mechanically to create and sustain vegetative existence. A person must be allowed dignified death. He must not be subjected to the doctor's death-fear or the relatives' harbored guilt. With our new medical technique a person should have increasing opportunity to elect time and manner of death. He should also have the chance to render his wishes to physician and family before he lapses into coma or goes into terminal illness where informed consent becomes impossible.

Socially, man must learn to die for the sake of the future. Here prespective ethical insight is strong. Global population and ecological disaster are imminent if we seek to disrupt the evolutionary death process now. We are already an octogenerically dominated society with a vicious generation crisis. The Senate records any day attest this. We must limit birth rate and maintain death rate if man is to survive on the planet. We are already dangerously close to that qualitatively bankrupt civilization predicted by Haldane where every human being is either sick, elderly, maimed, or working to care for such. We spend 10% of our GNP in this country on health. Although life energy is an important motivation, a visionary glimpse at our future should remind us of the ways this energy must be limited. We must learn again that death energy is creative.

Understood humanistically, death is that life event by which we pass on life to our children. Using the language of Elizabeth Kübler-Ross, we have created a unique biography; we have woven ourselves into the fabric of human history.[18] We can and generally do accept death with gratitude and contentment. Theologically understood, death signals the meaning of life in its conditionedness and contingency. It is God's ultimate attraction of our energy (Teilhard de Chardin).

Gideon is a marvelous expression of the interplay of life energy and the death impulse in divine-human affairs. It suffices as final illustration. Gideon has been commanded to slay the elders. But, being a man, he craves life. He disobeys the Lord and spares the elders. From the Lord's eternal perspective, man's thirst for existence is mildly rebellious folly and man's fear of death is amusing. The play ends with a moving yet paradoxical resolution of the theme we have explored in this chapter. Gideon is basking in the Lord's victory over the Midianites. He is tempted to deny its mystery and miracle and claim it as his own. Abimelech stares in awe at Gideon clad in the Lord's Golden vest.

Abimelech

We all wait to hear you tell the miracle of God's victory over Midiam.

Gideon

A miracle? Why do you call it that? My, my uncles, the war with Midian was not mysterious, but only the inevitable outgrowth of historico-economic, socio-psychological and cultural forces prevailing in these regions.

The Angel

Oh it is amusing.

God no more believes it odd
That man does not believe in God
Man believes the best he can
Which means, it seems, belief in man.
Then let him don my golden ephod
And let him be a proper God
Well, let him try it anyway
With this conceit, we end the play.[19]

# Postscript: The Future of Man:
# They Shall Be Like Gods . . .

We have begun the "final revolution." Through technology man's power is extended so that his activity defies simplistic, individualistic evaluation. He is technological man[1] and fabricated man.[2] His greatness and grandeur on the one hand and his failure and fall on the other will be accented in this development. Following matter and energy, human nature itself has come within the grasp of man's scientific and anticipatory intellect. Human reality will be increasingly drawn into the total objective world that man understands and controls.

Man is become like God. He possesses power to give and take life. In the Greek sense he has stolen knowledge, fire, and hope (insight, energy, and foresight) from the gods and now must learn to live responsibly with these powers. The history of his consciousness is marked with a religious perception and a humanistic urge. He has experienced the divine power as savior and judge, possibility and limitation. From pagan mythology he has been tantalized with the possibility of the death of God, the *Götterdämmerung* where the gods execute themselves out of being so that man can and must become God.

Responsibility entails faithfulness to both elements of consciousness. Man is godlike, but he is not God. His godlikeness creates in him immense capacities for knowledge and technology. It renders him responsible to constrain nature and human nature to ends as nobly conceived as his awareness permits. Yet he is no God. Death signals his frailty and more important his contingency. He belongs to a greater purpose. His tasks are but penultimate participations in that greater work, his constructions historical anticipations of that greater reality that transcends space and time.

This new power can serve his fulfillment or his destruction. The determination will be made on the basis of his wisdom, his insight, his foresight. This I have called retrospective, introspective, and prospective ethical perception.

The reader may perceive a theological bias in this book. I am searching for a new natural theology. I believe that man can discover as well as create value. I believe the cosmos to be a purposive process which signals through its inner dynamics its intrinsic ought. I believe man is made dynamically perceptive in memory, insight, and hope so that his mind can know and his will affirm that ever-emerging good which nature creates. I believe God is good. He is benevolent and beneficent creator. He has not deceptively or cruelly ordered nature but fashioned her vulnerable to man's perception and pliable to his will. This is not to deify or theomorphize man. Man is free under God. He can claim autonomy. He can will and accomplish destruction. He can corrupt self, nature, and history. The ethical imperatives thus arise with no inevitability but must be strongly posited, taught, nurtured, and protected in human life.

In all of the representative problems of biomedical ethics, we have seen this challenge. Man may use his mechanisms and technology for his liberation and fulfillment. He has profound sources of ethical insight at his disposal. Specific guidelines, directives, and intuitions must be sensitively worked out as one is responsive to the great moral energies of nature and the concrete decision-making situations in all their terrifying ambiguity. This book has attempted ethical theory. It has developed in somewhat erratic and inconsistent patterns. My philosopher colleagues will waste no time in calling this to my attention. Yet I have sought ethical insight into specific situations, concrete situations in medicine and technology. But I have sought to reflect on and evaluate these dynamic decision-making contexts. My clinical colleagues will justifiably question my abstraction. My hope is only that some few will take this book and find it instructive in that personal formation and living ethical perception that alone can save and heal this world.

# Notes

## Introduction

1. See Kenneth Vaux (ed.), *To Create a Different Future* (New York: Friendship Press, 1972).
2. Edward Kennedy, *In Critical Condition* (New York: Simon & Schuster, 1972).
3. Gerald Leach, *The Biocrats* (Baltimore: Penguin Books, 1972).
4. K. Danner Clouser, "Some Things Medical Ethics Is Not," in *Journal of the American Medical Association,* Vol. 223, No. 7 (Feb. 12, 1973), pp. 787–89.
5. The studies of Desmond Morris, *The Naked Ape* (New York: McGraw-Hill, 1968), Konrad Lorenz, *On Aggression* (New York: Harcourt Brace Jovanich, Inc., 1966), and Eugene Aubry, *The Territorial Imperative* (New York: Atheneum, 1966), are representative of this literature.
6. Abraham Heschel, *Who Is Man?* (Stanford: Stanford University Press, 1965), p. 22.
7. *Man a Machine* is the title of a famous work by La Mettrie (1709–51). An excellent analysis of the question of human nature explored in contrast to the machine is Mortimer Adler, *The Difference of Man and the Difference It Makes* (New York: Holt, Rinehart & Winston, 1967).
8. Hans Jonas, "Technology and Responsibility: Reflections on the New Tasks of Ethics," in *Journal of the American Academy of Religion* (Fall 1972), pp. 4 ff.

## The Hippocratic Tradition

1.  Paul Ramsey, *The Patient As Person* (New Haven: Yale University Press, 1970), p. ix.

2.  Asclepius, the principal god of healing in Greek religion after 300 B.C., apparently originated as a cultural hero called "The Blameless Old Physician" by Homer. Hygieia, it was said, was the daughter of Asclepius. On the Island of Cos in the fourth century B.C. there was a shrine to Asclepius. It was to the school of physicians on this island that Hippocrates belonged.

3.  The fact that god Apollo is invoked in the Hippocratic Oath has long puzzled scholars. That the gods had healing power was strongly believed. Perhaps Apollo was related to the healing mysteries associated with the Oracle of Delphi. In any case, a debate still wages concerning the religiomystical or secular origins of the Hippocratic tradition. Henry Sigerist in his *History of Medicine* argues, "The roots of Greek medical science and practice are to be sought not in temple lore but in the observations and thoughts of the early philosophers, and in the experience gained by trainers in the gymnasia." (New York: Oxford University Press, 1955, p. 45.)

4.  Although Ionian philosophy dealt principally with the sublimities of reality *(ta theia* and *ta meteora),* the great philosophers who precede the pre-Socratics begin turning attention to man *(ta anthropina).* The earliest and most influential school in this movement is the same order that shapes the Hippocratic medical ethos: the Pythagorean. The prime mover sought to avoid the flaws of mass society in the city-state and perfect a life-fulfilling discipline in small communities. The ideal of a sound mind in a sound body was pursued by a rigorous ritual which included diet, asceticism, mysticism, as well as the arts and crafts. Medicine, mathematics, and music were given a special place of prominence. If geometric numbers constituted the true essence of things, the craft of medicine yielded richer insight into truth than did the imprecise speculation of philosophy. To this day in medical education the basic wisdom that formed Hippocratic wisdom is normative. Man in his health and diseases is a fragment (microcosm) of the constitution of the world and can be understood only *sub specie* of this macrocosm. See in

this regard the excellent monograph W. H. S. Jones, *Philosophy and Medicine in Ancient Greece* (Baltimore: The Johns Hopkins University Press, 1946).

5.  The focus in Hippocratic tradition was on the healthy balance of life. Alcmaeon, the prototype of the Hippocratic physician, reflected on health in this way:

> "Health is a condition maintained by equality *(isonomia)* among the powers, the moist, the dry, the cold, the hot, the bitter, the sweet and the rest, but an autocracy *(monarchia)* among these produces disease. . . . Health is an harmonious blending of the various qualities. . . . A mixture *(krasis)* of opposing energies *(dunameis)*."

Ibid., pp. 6 ff.

6.  One of the most brilliant statements of this optimism in Greek thought is found in Diogenes Laertius (VIII 59: Hicks translation) which records the view of the Empedoclean school which deeply influenced the Hippocratic outlook. The world view expresses optimism in the power of man ultimately to control all the vitalities of nature. It is not unlike the New Testament confidence that faith can move mountains.

> "Thou shalt learn all the drugs that are a defense to ward off ills and old age, since for thee alone shall I accomplish all this. Thou shalt arrest the violence of the unwearied winds that arise and sweep the earth, laying waste the cornfields with their blasts; and again, if thou so will, though shalt call back winds in requital. Thou shalt make after the dark rain a seasonable drought for men, and again after the summer drought thou shalt cause tree-nourishing streams to pour from the sky. Thou shalt bring back from Hades a dead man's strength."

Ibid., p. 11, 12.

7.  Ramsey, op. cit., p. 97.
8.  Erik Erikson, "Protest and Affirmation," in *Harvard Medical Bulletin* (Fall 1972), p. 31.
9.  Sigerist, op. cit., pp. 238–40.
10. Jones, op. cit., p. 16.

## The Religious Traditions

1. A recent joint meeting of the American Association for the Advancement of Science and the Mexican counterpart (Consejo Nacional de Ciencia y Tecnología) evidenced to this author the vapid inadequacy of most American protagonists especially when contrasted with some Latin Americans of Marxist persuasion. On the issues of concern for defective children and care for the humanizing of the dying person, the attitudinal contrast was very evident. At this particular meeting Dr. William May, chairman of the religion department at Indiana University, commented on the similarity in emphasis between the papers of Dr. Eric Cassell (U.S.A.) and Luis Weinstein (Chile). In discussing the problem both called on extrinsic values to enlighten bare technological aspects of death in a clinical setting. Cassell invoked the distinction between the moral and technical dimension and Weinstein argued the importance of the socio-ethical reality.

JUDAISM:

1. See Kenneth Vaux, "Technology and the Human Quest" (yet unpublished manuscript). In this work I argue that the vision of a righteous kingdom in Judaic hope fundamentally constitutes our quest for an unambiguous future.

2. Emmanuel Jacobovits, *Jewish Medical Ethics: A Comparative Study of the Jewish Religions* (New York: Bloch Publishing Co., 1962), and David Feldman, *Birth Control in Jewish Law* (New York: New York University Press, 1968).

3. I emphasize the salvific aspects of Hebrew understanding because this is the theological backdrop for the elaborations of the law which are found in Torah and the derivative ethical material in the Talmud, Mishna, Responsa, and other teaching. The casuistry (Rabbi Hillel said . . . ) is always presented as the reason for specific medico-moral guidelines and one is not always cognizant of the rich theological foundation for the moral insight.

4. See for example Solomon B. Freehof, "Death and Burial in the Jewish Tradition," in Daniel Jeremy Silver (ed.), *Judaism and Ethics* (New York: KTAV Publishing House, 1970), pp. 201 ff.

5. Abraham Heschel, *Who Is Man* (Stanford: Stanford University Press, 1965), p. 41.

ISLAM:

1. Martin Levey, "Medical Ethics of Medieval Islam with Special Reference to Al-Ruhāwis' Practical Ethics of the Physician," in *Transactions of the American Philosophical Society* (Philadelphia: APS Press, 1967), Vol. 57, Part 3, pp. 13 ff.
2. Ibid., pp. 70–71.

ROMAN CATHOLICISM:

1. Gerald Kelly, *Medico-Moral Problems* (St. Louis: Catholic Hospital Association, 1958). Edwin F. Healy, *Medical Ethics* (Chicago: Loyola University Press, 1960).
2. Healy, ibid., pp. 184, 185.

PROTESTANTISM:

1. James Gustafson has provided the basis for his medico-moral thought in *Christ and the Moral Life* (New York: Harper & Row, 1968) and *Christian Ethics and the Community* (Philadelphia: Pilgrim Press, 1971). His more recent writing has focused on the medical field. Most papers are privately distributed documents of the Hastings Institute, Hastings-on-Hudson, New York.
2. André Dumas, the brilliant French Protestant, stands in the circle of provocative thinkers including Roger Mehl and Jacques Ellul. The book *Prospective et Prophétie* (Paris: du Cerf, 1972) is his first treatment of these problems.
3. Paul Ramsey has contributed both general analysis and specified studies to the literature of medical ethics. *Deeds and Rule in Christian Ethics* (New York: Scribner's, 1967) and *Basic Christian Ethics* (New York: Scribner's, 1950) illustrate the former. Problem-focused writing includes *Fabricated Man: The Genetic Control* (New Haven: Yale University Press, 1970) and *The Patient As Person* (New Haven: Yale University Press, 1970).
4. Paul Ramsey, "The Case of the Curious Exception," in Gene Outka and Paul Ramsey (eds.), *Norm and Context in Christian Ethics* (New York: Scribner's, 1968), p. 123.
5. Joseph Fletcher has lifted medicomoral issues to the forefront of

public consciousness for many years. His pertinent titles are: *Morals and Medicine* (Boston: Beacon Press, 1960), *Moral Responsibility* (Philadelphia: Westminster Press, 1967), *Situation Ethics* (Philadelphia: Westminster Press, 1966), and a new study on Genetic Ethics soon to be released by Doubleday.

6. Joseph Fletcher, "What's in a Rule: A Situationist's View," in Gene Outka and Paul Ramsey (eds.), *Norm and Context in Christian Ethics* (New York: Scribner's, 1968), p. 342.

7. Daniel Callahan, "Bioethics As a Discipline," in *The Hastings Center Studies,* Vol. 1, No. 1 (1973), p. 70.

8. Joseph Fletcher, "Criteria for Personhood," a yet unpublished paper which is summarized in *The Hastings Center Report,* Vol. 2, No. 5 (Nov. 1972).

9. Dietrich Bonhoeffer, *Ethics* (New York: Macmillan, 1965).

10. Karl Barth, *Church Dogmatics* (Edinburgh: T & T Clark, 1961).

11. In addition to his principal literature, *Theologische Ethik* Bände I-III (Tübingen: J. Mohr, 1960), English translation, *Theological Ethics* (Philadelphia: Fortress Press, 1970), the reader is referred to a small study *Der Artz als Richter: Wer Darf Leben?* (Tübingen: Rainer Wunderlich Verlag Hermann Leins, 1968). This monograph is translated and included in the volume by Kenneth Vaux (ed.), *Who Shall Live?* (Philadelphia: Fortress Press, 1970). *The Ethics of Sex* (New York: Harper & Row, 1964) is essentially a review of the corresponding section in the *Ethik.*

12. Helmut Thielicke, *Theologische Ethik II, 1.2* (Tübingen: J. Mohr, 1958).

13. Michael Hemphill, "Pretesting for Huntington's Disease," in *The Hastings Center Report,* Vol. 3, No. 3 (June 1973), pp. 12 ff.

**MARXISM:**

1. In his 1970 Gifford Lectures Aarend Th. van Leeuwen argues that Marx's thought has a "profoundly theological character." His "Critique of Heaven" is accompanied by a "Critique of the Earth" within which man is affirmed and religion recalled to its essential task of humanizing the earth. Aarend Th. van Leeuwen, *Critique of Heaven* (New York: Scribner's, 1973), p. 24.

## The Neuremberg Tradition

1.  William L. Shirer, *The Rise and Fall of the Third Reich* (Greenwich, Conn.: Fawcett Books, 1960), pp. 1274 ff.
2.  Ibid., p. 1274.
3.  A. Mitscherlich and F. Mielke, *Doctors of Infamy* (New York: Henry Schuman, 1949), p. 200.
4.  Lawrence Kohlberg, "The Development of Modes of Moral Thinking and Choice in the Years 10 to 16" (Chicago: University of Chicago Thesis Photocopy, 1969).
5.  Henry Beecher, *Research and the Individual: Human Studies* (Boston: Little, Brown & Company, 1970), pp. 229 ff.

## A Model for Decision-making

1.  Immanuel Kant, *Foundations of the Metaphysics of Morals* (New York: Bobbs-Merrill Co., Inc., 1959). See also David Ross, *Kant's Ethical Theory: A Commentary on the Grundlegung zur Metaphysik der Sitten* (Oxford: The Clarendon Press, 1954); Josef Santeler, *Die Grundlegung der Menschenwürde bei I. Kant* (Innsbruck: AMCE Press, 1962); and J. W. Scott, *Kant on the Moral Life: An Exposition of Kant's Grundlegung* (London: A. & C. Black, Ltd., 1924).
2.  John Rawls, *A Theory of Justice* (Cambridge, Mass.: Harvard University Press, 1971).
3.  Ibid., pp. 14, 15.
4.  Wolfhart Pannenberg, *Theology of the Kingdom of God* (Philadelphia: Westminster Press, 1969), p. 73.

## Generating Man

1.  One of our medical colleges has the policy of mandatory screening for sickle-cell anemia for employees and students of the Institution. Although the possibilities of "on the job" crisis are not so great for carriers as for those afflicted with the disease, they were isolated in the screening. The problems of informing, bearing responsibility for the information, providing genetic counseling, were immediately raised. As Robert Mur-

ray and Marc Lappe have pointed out, we should be absolutely certain we can bear the consequences of our knowledge and technology in this area. See Robert Murray, "Ethical and Moral Aspects of Genetic Knowledge and Counseling," in Kenneth Vaux (ed.), *To Create a Different Future* (New York: Friendship Press, 1972), pp. 67 ff. Marc Lappe, "How Much Do We Want to Know About the Unborn?" in *The Hastings Center Report,* Vol. 3 No. 1 (Feb. 1973), pp. 8, 9.

2.  "Service Diagnoses Birth Defects Early," in *Atlanta Constitution,* July 9, 1973, p. 413.

3.  Robert Sinsheimer, "Prospects for Future Scientific Developments: Ambush or Opportunity," in Daniel Callahan and Bruce Hilton et al. (eds.). *Ethical Issues in Human Genetics* (New York: Plenum Press, 1973).

4.  Carlo Valenti, "Antenatal Detection of Hemoglobinopathies: A Preliminary Report," in *American Journal of Obstetrics and Gynecology,* Vol. 115, No. 6 (Mar. 15, 1973), pp. 851–53.

5.  Albert Rosenfeld, *The Second Genesis: The Coming Control of Life* (Englewood Cliffs, N.J.: Prentice-Hall, 1969).

6.  David M. Rorvik, "Making Men and Women Without Men and Women," in *Esquire,* Apr. 1969, pp. 108 ff.

7.  Sinsheimer, op. cit., p. 341.

8.  Paul Ramsey, "Shall We Clone a Man?" in Kenneth Vaux (ed.), *Who Shall Live?* (Philadelphia: Fortress Press, 1970), pp. 77 ff.

9.  Shamai Kanter, "If Man Creates Life Is He Still Man?" in *National Jewish Monthly,* Nov. 1963.

10. Ian Barbour, *Science and Secularity* (New York: Harper & Row, 1970), pp. 76 ff.

11. Richard Kaufman, "Quest for the 'Superman': Modern Man and Biology," in Egbert de Vries (ed.), *Man in Community* (New York: Association Press, 1966), pp. 218 ff.

12. Herman Muller, "Our Load by Mutations," in *American Journal of Human Genetics* 11, 2 (June 1950); "The Guidance of Human Evolution," in *Perspectives in Biology and Medicine,* III (Autumn 1959), University of Chicago, 1959; "Means and Aims in Human Genetic Betterment," in Tracy M. Sonneborn (ed.), *The Control of Human Heredity and Evolution* (New York: Macmillan, 1965); "Better Genes for Tomorrow," in Stuart Mudd (ed.), *The Population Crisis and the Use*

*of World Resources* (The Hague: Dr. W. Junk Publishers, 1964); see also H. J. Muller, Bibliography.

13. See for example the testimony of Joshua Lederberg on Senate Joint Resolution 145 for the establishment of the National Commission on Health, Science and Society (Washington: Committee on Government Operations, 1968), pp. 54 ff.

14. Margery W. Shaw, Principal Discussant of F. Clarke Fraser, "Survey of Counseling Practices," in Daniel Callahan and Bruce Hilton et al. (eds.), op. cit., pp. 13–17.

15. See for example Muller, "The Guidance of Human Evolution," in op. cit., p. 11, where he states that a future society of "hopeless," utterly diverse genetic monstrosities will result if we proceed with present understanding. This will create a situation where population is constituted largely by the "lame and weak," where "the job of ministering to infirmities would come to consume all the energy that society could muster." For commentary on the ethical context of this "genetic apocalypse" see Paul Ramsey, "Moral and Religious Implications of Genetic Control," in John Roslansky (ed.), *Genetics and the Future of Man* (New York: Appleton-Century-Crofts, 1966), pp. 132–34. Helmut Thielicke comments on this concern in his essay "The Doctor As Judge of Who Shall Live" in Kenneth Vaux (ed.), *Who Shall Live?*, op. cit., pp. 146 ff.

16. See for example Bernard Haring, *The Law of Christ* (Westminster, Md.: Newman, 1966), pp. 73 ff.

17. Immanuel Jakobovits, *Jewish Medical Ethics* (New York: Bloch Publishing Co., 1959), pp. 154–55; for additional Jewish theological references to the themes of procreation, see Jacobovits, ch. 13–15, also Bibliography.

18. Paul Ramsey, "Moral and Religious Implications of Genetic Control," in John Roslansky (ed.), op. cit., p. 147.

19. Helmut Thielicke, *Theologische Ethik: Band III* (Tübingen: J. C. B. Mohr (Paul Siebeck, 1964), pp. 507 ff. An abbreviated English edition of Thielicke's Sexuality Ethic is available in *Ethics of Sex* (New York: Harper & Row, 1964).

20. William Pollard, *Man on a Spaceship* (Claremont, Calif.: The Claremont Colleges, 1967), p. 20.

21. Ramsey, op. cit., pp. 149–50.

22. Gerhard Von Rad, *Genesis* (Philadelphia: Westminster Press, 1961), pp. 55–59.

23. Pierre Teilhard de Chardin, *Building the Earth* (Wilkes-Barre, Pa.: Dimension Books, 1965), p. 75.

24. Margaret Mead, "The Cultural Shaping of the Ethical Context," in *Who Shall Live?* Kenneth Vaux (ed.), op. cit., p. 10.

25. Dag Hammarskjöld, *Markings* (New York: Alfred A. Knopf, 1964), p. xvi.

26. Daniel Callahan, *Abortion: Law Choice and Morality* (New York: Macmillan, 1971), Introduction.

27. Pearl Buck, quoted in *The Terrible Choice: The Abortion Dilemma* (New York: Bantam Books, 1968), p. x.

## Rebuilding Man

1. D. A. Cooley, D. Liotta, G. L. Hallman, R. D. Bloodwell, R. D. Leachman and J. D. Milam, "First Human Implantation of Cardiac Prosthesis for Staged Total Replacement of the Heart," in *Transaction of the American Society of Artificial Internal Organs,* Vol. 15 (1969), pp. 252–64.

2. See for example "Cardiac Replacement: Medical, Ethical, Psychological and Economic Implications," in *Report of AD HOC Task Force of Cardiac Replacement,* National Heart Institute, Oct. 1969, recommendations pp. 61, 62 (Washington, D. C., U. S. Department of Health, Education and Welfare).

3. The "hyperacute rejection reaction" of the heterograft probably rules out increased use of this procedure until immunosuppressive knowledge increased. See N. H. I. "cardiac Replacement . . ." report, op. cit., p. 25.

4. The complex dialectics of freedom and coercion are vivid under these circumstances. The siblings (ideally the identical twin) know they are the most desirable donor when brother or sister needs a kidney.

5. "The Ultimate Operation," in *Time,* Dec. 15, 1967, p. 64.

6. For an excellent account of this procedure and the broad social activity it represents, see Renee Fox and Judith Swazey, *The Courage to Fail: Transplantation on Man* (Chicago: University of Chicago Press, 1973).

7.  "Transplants: Summit for the Heart," in *Time*, July 26, 1968, p. 50.

8.  Irvin Kraft, "Clinical Psychiatric Aspects of a Cardiac Transplantation Program," p. 6. This paper supplied by the author will be published at a later stage.

9.  Ibid., p. 8.

10. See Kenneth Vaux, "Ethical Dimensions of the Heart Transplant," in *Christian Century*, Vol. LXXXV, No. 12 (Mar. 20, 1968), p. 354.

11. Ibid., p. 354 (the Darvall family reaction). Kraft, op. cit., p. 15, also notes the clear religious conviction in donor families that the deceased lives on in the recipient either in the extension of life granted or in immortality.

12. Ruth Nanda Anshen, *Freedom: Its Meaning* (New York: Harcourt Brace and Co., 1940), p. 6.

13. D. S. Halacy, Jr., *Cyborg: Evolution of the Superman* (New York: Harper & Row, 1965). Halacy's discussion of the heart replacement begins on p. 75.

14. Carl F. Henry, "Are Heart Transplants Moral?" editorial in *Christianity Today*, Feb. 16, 1968, p. 502.

15. Dietrich Bonhoeffer, *Letters and Papers from Prison* (London: Fontana Books, 1953), p. 50.

16. These statements are based on my interviews with hospital chaplains who have counseled with heart transplant patients. Although nothing is published on this, the experience of the Reverend Arman Jorjorian and his chaplain corps at St. Luke's in Houston has been most helpful. The proceedings from the *First International Symposium on Medico-Social Aspects of Organ Transplantation* (privately distributed document at St. Luke's Hospital, Houston) contains material on this point.

17. The living bank in Houston and the Los Angeles organ pool are donation programs where the altruistic commitment is the essence of the appeal. See for example my article, "A Year of Heart Transplants: An Ethical Evaluation," in *Journal of Postgraduate Medicine*, Vol. 45, No. 1 (Jan. 1969), p. 203. See also the *Los Angeles Times* article by Harry Nelson, "Los Angeles Doctors Form Pool for Organs for Transplants," Jan. 9, 1968, p. 1.

18. A big step in this direction has been made by the adoption in forty states of the uniform anatomical gift act. See A. M. Sadler and B. L. Sadler,

"Transplantation and the Law: The Need for Organized Sensitivity," in *Georgetown Law Journal* Vol. 57 (1967), pp. 5–54.

19. Vaux, in *Postgraduate Medicine,* op. cit., p. 201.

20. Henry Beecher, "Prepared Statement for the Hearings on the Establishment of a National Commission on Health, Science and Society," in *Committee on Government Operations* (Washington: U. S. Printing Office, 1968), p. 108.

21. Joshua Lederberg, *Committee on Government Operations,* op. cit., p. 54. The problem that Lederberg calls "The Heart Gap," i.e., needy recipients outnumbering possible donors, is one exposed clearly in the media announcement of these events.

22. "Cardiac Replacement," in *N. H. I. Study,* op. cit., p. 42.

23. Irvin Kraft, op. cit., pp. 14, 15.

24. H. Richard Niebuhr, *The Responsible Self* (New York: Harper & Row, 1964), p. 126.

25. Theodosius Dobzhansky, "Human Values in an Evolving World," in Cameron P. Hall (ed.), *Human Values and Advancing Technology* (New York: Friendship Press, 1968), p. 67.

## Controlling Man

1. Aldous Huxley, *Brave New World* (New York: Bantam Books, 1954).

2. B. F. Skinner, *Beyond Freedom and Dignity* (New York: Knopf, 1971).

3. Michael Crichton, *The Terminal Man* (New York: Knopf, 1972).

4. Albert Rosenfeld, *The Second Genesis: The Coming Control of Life* (Englewood Cliffs, N. J.: Prentice-Hall, 1969).

5. Arthur Koestler's study of *The Ghost in the Machine* (New York: Macmillan, 1967) points out the self-destructive tendencies in man which are heightened in technology. His *Darkness at Noon* (New York: Macmillan, 1941) was one of the first works to remind the English-speaking world of the psychosocial terror of mind control.

6. Good introduction to the three aspects of mind manipulation are found in Seymour M. Farber and Robert H. L. Wilson (eds.), *Control of the Mind* (New York: McGraw-Hill, 1961); Jose Delgado, *Physical Control of the Mind: Toward a Psychocivilized Society* (New York: Harper & Row, 1970), and Albert Rosenfeld, op. cit.

7. Marshall McLuhan, *Understanding Media: The Extensions of Man* (New York: McGraw-Hill, 1964).

8. Pierre Teilhard de Chardin, *The Phenomenon of Man* (New York: Harper Torchbooks, 1959).

9. The classic formulation of the rational nature of mind and reality and the microcosmic/macrocosmic relation of man's reason and nature is found in *The Republic of Plato*.

10. Albert Moraczewski, "The Divorce of Psyche and Soma," in *Psychosomatics*, Vol. 11, No. 3 (May-June 1970), pp. 151 in ff.

11. Emil Brunner, *Man in Revolt* (Philadelphia: Westminster Press, 1939).

12. Expressions of this point were many and varied in the literature. See for example Martin Buber, *I and Thou* (New York: Scribner's, 1958); Karl Barth, *Church Dogmatics III*, 2, 45 (Edinburgh: T. & T. Clark, 1956), and Helmut Thielicke, *The Ethics of Sex*, translated by John W. Doberstein (New York: Harper & Row, 1964).

13. Jan Kamaryt, "Principles of the Marxist Understanding of Man and Humanism," in Hans Rudi Weber (ed.), *Experiments with Man* (Geneva: World Council of Churches, 1969), pp. 68–69.

14. Roger Garaudy, *From Anathema to Dialogue* (New York: Vintage, 1968).

15. Kenneth Vaux, "A Year of Heart Transplants: An Ethical Evaluation," in *Journal of Postgraduate Medicine*, Vol. 45, No. 1 (Jan. 1969).

16. H. Richard Niebuhr, *The Responsible Self* (New York: Harper & Row, 1964), p. 126.

17. Rosenfeld, op. cit., p. 190.

18. For a discussion of the meaning of intentionality see Rollo May, *Love and Will* (New York: Norton Books, 1969).

19. Jose Delgado, "Brain Technology and Psychocivilization," in Cameron Hall (ed.), *Human Values and Advancing Technology*, (New York: Friendship Press, 1968). This paper is a slightly modified version of talk given at the Columbia University Seminars on Technology and Social Change, Nov. 10, 1966.

20. See Kenneth Vaux, "Statement before the Subcommittee on Government Research," Hearings on S. J. Resolution 145. To establish a National Commission on Health, Science and Society, Washington, D. C., 1968, p. 138.

21. Ibid., p. 138.
22. Delgado, op. cit., p. 81.
23. See Norbert Wiener, *The Human Use of Human Beings* (Boston: Houghton Mifflin Company, 1954).
24. Karl Rahner, "Christianity and the New Earth," in Walter J. Ong (ed.), *Knowledge and the Future of Man* (New York: Holt, Rinehart & Winston, 1968), p. 268.

## Immortalizing Man

1. Paddy Chayefsky, *Gideon* (New York: Random House, 1961), p. 99.
2. David Bakan, *Disease, Pain and Sacrifice* (Chicago: University of Chicago Press, 1968).
3. Violent rejection invariably occurs in cross-species tissue grafts. The desperation attempt to transplant a ram's heart into a human being resulted in hyperacute rejection (Denton A. Cooley et al., "Human Heart Transplantation Experience with Twelve Cases," in *The American Journal of Cardiology*, Vol. 22, No. 6 [Dec. 1968], p. 810). Reflection on the first xenograft is presented in the clinical report of James D. Hardy who transplanted the heart of a chimpanzee into a human being. James D. Hardy and Carlos M. Chavez, "The First Heart Transplant in Man: Developmental Animal Investigations with Analysis of the 1964 Case in the Light of Current Clinical Experience," in *The American Journal of Cardiology*, Vol. 22, No. 6 (Dec. 1968), pp. 272 ff.
4. "Bench Surgery Being Perfected for Human Use," in *Baylor Medicine Review*, Vol. 1, No. 1 (Spring 1971), p. 22.
5. Dylan Thomas, *Collected Poems* (New York: New Directions, 1952), p. 150.
6. Henry Beecher et al., "A Definition of Irreversible Coma," in *Journal of the American Medical Association*, Vol. 205, No. 6 (Aug. 5, 1968), pp. 337 ff.
7. Tone Kvittingen and A. Naess, "Recovery from Drowning in Fresh Water," in *British Medical Journal*, May 18, 1963.
8. Nikolai Amosoff, *Notes from the Future* (New York: Simon & Schuster, 1970), p. 101.
9. Ibid., p. 207.
10. Ibid., p. 303.

11. Ibid., pp. 291–92.
12. "Notes from the Future," in *Look*, Aug. 14, 1970, p. 58.
13. Amosoff, op. cit., p. 317.
14. Herman Kahn and Anthony J. Wiener, *The Year 2000* (New York: Macmillan, 1967), pp. 53 ff.
15. *Look*, op. cit., p. 65.
16. Robert C. W. Ettinger, *The Prospect of Immortality* (New York: Mac-Fadden Books, 1964), pp. 75–76 (*my additions).
17. Kenneth Vaux, "A Year of Heart transplants: An Ethical Valuation," in *Postgraduate Medicine*, Vol. 45, No. 1 (January, 1969), pp. 204, 205.
18. Elizabeth Kübler-Ross, *On Death and Dying* (New York: Macmillan, 1969), p. 277.
19. Paddy Chaeysky, op. cit., p. 108. a

## Postscript

1. Victor Ferkiss, *Technological Man: The Myth and the Reality* (New York: Braziller Co., 1970).
2. Paul Ramsey, *Fabricated Man* (New Haven: Yale University Press, 1970).

# Glossary

Amniocentesis: a technique by which a small amount of amniotic fluid is removed from the uterus during gestation for examination and diagnosis of certain congenital defects or diseases prior to the birth of the baby.

Android systems: machines built from hardware and software that take on the likeness of man.

Arteriosclerotic: the building up of fatty cells on the intravascular walls. The encrustation combined with hardening and lesions is a major condition of cardiovascular illness.

Biocybernetics: the discipline of applying feedback models of analysis to living systems.

Cloning: the process of replicating from one simple healthy cell an organism identical to the one from which the cell was taken. The process occurs by denucleating an egg cell and nucleating it with the nucleus of the organism one desires to clone.

Conscience: the sensibility in man by which he perceives his possibility and responsibility. The perception activates guilt or dissatisfaction when one misses the mark.

Cryobiology: the science inquiring into the effect of low temperature and freezing on various forms of life. Cryogenics, cryosurgery, and human hibernation are human activities related to this discipline.

Cyborg: the joining to human life of an artificial substance or apparatus to modify the functioning of that person.

Cytogenetic analysis: the technique of analyzing fetal cells to detect chromosome characteristics. The test gives indications of inherited abnormalities.

Ecosphere: the total environment of all life wherein all systems interact and thus affect each other in the interaction. Man, the other animals and plants as well as the barysphere, hydrosphere, atmosphere, lithosphere, are comprehended in this total environment.

Endoamnioscopy: a new technique developed to diagnose a fetus antenatally. The instrument first described by Dr. Carlos Valenti (*American Journal of Obstetrics and Gynecology*, Vol. 115, No. 6, March 15, 1973, pp. 851–53) takes a sample of blood and tissue from the fetus and makes available a wide profile of characteristics.

Euthanasia: a good death. The common meaning of the term implies positive interventions or restraints from interventions that facilitate easy death in one suffering in extremis.

Extrauterine gestation: the process of nurturing a developing organism in laboratory facilities outside the womb of the mother.

Hemochromatosis: a rare hereditable disease characterized by uncontrollable absorption of dietary iron.

Hemodialysis: the mechanical process of cleaning and processing blood when there is partial or complete kidney shutdown. The technique is often preliminary to renal transplantation.

Homotransplantation: the implantation of tissue from an organism of the same species. This is distinguished from heterotransplantation, where the donor is of another species, and autotransplantation, where tissue is retrieved from other tissues of the same organism.

Huntington's disease (Huntington's Chorea): a hereditary disease characterized by shaking choreic movements and mental deterioration. The disease usually has symptomatic onset between ages 30 and 50.

Hypothermia: decreased body temperature in an organism as a result of internal or external forces.

Informed consent: a fundamental criterion in medical ethics whereby a recipient of a given procedure is given all relevant knowledge and expected to show comprehension of that knowledge to the attending professional. The connotation of education as the essence of informed consent is given widespread acceptance.

K tenology: the science of killing. The term gained wide coinage during Nazi medicine experiments and subsequent trials. In those cases therapeutic and even scientific value was suspended in pursuit of the value of inflicting death.

Negative eugenics: the science of breeding out or offsetting the effect of deleterious traits in offspring.

PKU: an inborn error of metabolism characterized by elevation of blood phenylalanine frequently associated with mental retardation.

Positive eugenics: the science of building in or reinforcing positive traits in offspring. Methods include selective breeding as well as direct modification of germinal material. Donor insemination is an important technique pursuant of this goal.

Sickle cell anemia: a chronic disease endemic to Blacks, wherein the red blood cells become sickle-shaped, creating anemia and early death. Ten percent of Blacks carry the trait.

Spina bifida: congenital defect of the spinal column involving bifurcation which affects the spinal cord. The child normally has no neural response in the lower trunk.

Tay Sachs disease: the infantile form of amaurotic familial idiocy, a degenerative disorder which results in progressive degeneration of cerebral function characterized by dementia, paralysis, epilepsy, and blindness. The disease is fatal and rarely extends beyond the fifth year. It is common to Ashkenazic Jews.

Tetraparental Chimera: an organism formed by mixing the germinal material of four different parents. Experimentation has also occurred using parentage of different species.

Trunk prosthesis: in treating a hemicorporectomy patient (excising the legs and lower parts of the upper body), a carriage is built into which the upper half of the body is placed.

# INDEX

abortion, 23, 25, 43, 50, 51, 58, 65–68
amniocentesis, 9, 23, 50, 51, 58, 64–65
artificial organs, 99
autotransplantation, 99

behavior control, 87
  socio-political organs of control, xvii–
    xviii, 87–88
  technical manipulation of the brain,
    87–88
brain death, 102

cloning, 51–52, 60–61
common sense, 41, 43
conscience, 17, 20, 38, 39, 42, 43, 89
covenant, 5–6, 11, 14, 18, 42, 63
creativity, 55–60
cryogenics, 104–105
  cryosurgery, 106
  ethical issues, 105–107
  hibernation and evolution, 106

death and dying, 21, 97–113
death impulse, 101
decision-making, xv, xviii, 37–45
dignity of man, xvi

ecology, xiv, 44
euthanasia, 20

fall of man, 22, 53
fidelity, 6

Fletcher, Joseph, 20–21
freedom, 17, 66, 76, 80, 81–82, 89–91,
  93

genetic alteration, 49–68

health, ix
heart transplant, x, 70–76
  artificial heart, 77, 80–83
Hippocratic tradition, 3–9
  in Neuremberg code, 27
humanism, 31–32, 38, 55

informed consent, 31, 76, 81
Islam, 13–14

Judaism, 11–13, 39–40, 61–62
life as a gift, 12, 18, 23
life impulse, 97–101
life prolongation, 9
love, 5, 18–20, 23, 39, 62, 79, 93

man and animal life, xiii
man and machine, xiv, xv
man as a creature of God, 12, 39–40,
  55–56
man as a whole
  health as wholeness, 8–9
  in Hippocratic tradition, 7–8
Marxism, 24–25, 90–91
medical students, xi–xiii
medicine and society

in Marxism, 24–25
in Neuremberg, 26–27

natural law
in Catholicism, 16
in Protestantism, 17
Neuremberg code, 12, 21, 29–32, 40
Neuremberg tradition, 26–33

"playing God," 54
procreativity, 60–68
Protestantism, 17–24, 61–62, 90

Ramsey, Paul, 3, 17–19, 55, 62–63
relatedness and community, 63, 108
Roman Catholicism, 14–17, 61, 90

Socrates, 5
technology, x–xi, xv, xvii–xviii
Thielicke, Helmut, 22–24, 62
transplantation, x, 69, 98–101

will of God, 92